Clinical and Laboratory Performance of

BONE PLATES

Harvey/Games, editors

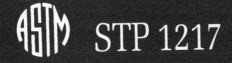 STP 1217

STP 1217

Clinical and Laboratory Performance of Bone Plates

J. Paul Harvey, Jr. and Robert F. Games, editors

ASTM Publication Code Number (PCN)
04-012170-54

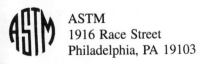

ASTM
1916 Race Street
Philadelphia, PA 19103

Library of Congress Cataloging-in-Publication Data

Clinical laboratory performance of bone plates / J. Paul Harvey, Jr.
and Robert F. Games. editors.
    (STP ; 1217)
    Includes bibliographical references and index.
    ISBN 0-8031-1897-X
    1. Bone plates (Orthopedics)--Testing--Congresses. 2. Internal
fixation in fractures--Congresses.   I. Harvey, J. Paul, 1922-
II. Games, Robert F. III. Series: ASTM special technical
publication ; 1217.
    [DNLM: 1. Bone Plates--congresses. 2. Bone Screws--congresses.
3. Materials Testing--methods--congresses. 4. Fracture Fixation,
Internal--instrumentation--congresses.   WE 185 C641 1994]
RD103.I5C56 1994
617.1'5--dc20
DNLM/DLC
for Library of Congress   93-49642
                                                                  CIP

Photocopy Rights

Peer Review Policy

Each paper published in this volume was evaluated by three peer reviewers. The authors
addressed all of the reviewers' comments to the satisfaction of both the technical editor(s) and
the ASTM Committee on Publications.

To make technical information available as quickly as possible, the peer-reviewed papers in
this publication were printed "camera-ready" as submitted by the authors.

The quality of the papers in this publication reflects not only the obvious efforts of the authors
and the technical editor(s), but also the work of these peer reviewers. The ASTM Committee
on Publications acknowledges with appreciation their dedication and contribution to time and
effort on behalf of ASTM.

Printed in Philadelphia, PA

February 1994

Foreword

This publication, *Clinical and Laboratory Performance of Bone Plates*, contains papers presented at the symposium of the same name, held in Atlanta, GA on 5 May 1993. The symposium was sponsored by ASTM Committee F-4 on Surgical Materials and Devices. J. Paul Harvey, Jr. of Pasadena, CA and Robert F. Games of Smith & Nephew Richards, Inc. in Memphis, TN presided as symposium chairmen and are editors of the resulting publication.

Contents

CLINICAL APPLICATION

Overview

This manual is the result of a symposium on clinical and laboratory performance of bone plates, organized by Committee F-4 of ASTM, in an effort to stimulate the production of new standards for the clinical performance of bone plates. The standards for design of bone plates and standards for laboratory testing of bone plates are in existence, but neither type of standard takes into account clinical performance, which is the *raison d'etre* of these plates.

One major difficulty in writing performance standards is that when we clinicians are asked what stress and strain occurs in anatomical bones and what strength and stiffness should manufacturers provide in apparatus used to maintain fixation of fractures in these bones, we have no specific answers. When a fracture occurs, we ordinarily try to reduce the fracture and maintain a reduction by immobilizing the bone by some device such as plaster of Paris cast, external fixation device, plates attached to the bones by screws, or an intramedullary rod, or perhaps other means. We then immobilize the area by a plaster of Paris cast or a splint of some type to prevent motion of the bones involved, which means immobilizing the joints above (proximal) and below (distal) to the fracture. Most function of the bone is prevented by these measures, but not all. Some motion beyond the area fixed will cause muscle activity acting on the immobilized area. Fractured bones in the lower extremity are usually prevented from weight-bearing by the use of crutches, wheelchair, or bed rest for varying periods of time. If the clinician thinks that the fixation device is strong enough and there is preferably total contact of the bone fragments, one may not immobilize the area at all, particularly in the upper extremities, and may allow early weight-bearing in the lower extremities. Therefore, it becomes apparent that the clinician will be helped by understanding the meaning and significance of the numbers provided by bioengineers and manufacturers in relationships to the tests done on the devices, particularly plates, provided by manufacturers and engineers. Conversely, it is important that engineers and manufacturers should understand the problems facing the clinician and the amount of his knowledge, or lack of knowledge, about the factors affecting these problems in a clinical setting.

Obviously, if the clinician knew the exact forces and their directions when applied to bones as function occurs, engineers and manufacturers could simply provide a device whose strength, easily determined by tests, would be sufficient to counteract the forces applied. In the instance of plates, fixation to the bone has not been considered, but screws are commonly used to hold the plate in place. The plate must be of such a design as to fit or be bent to fit the anatomy for bone involved, and be of such a size as to fit easily within the elastic soft tissue envelope covering the bone in question. Plates as well as screws used to fix fractures in bones in the hand and finger are obviously different in size in all dimensions from the plate used to fix fractures of the femur. The plates may also be attached to intramedullary devices at one end, such as an intramedullary nail (for the femoral neck) or an intramedullary blade for fixation, particularly but not only of the ends of the femur.

Many other factors enter into the performance of bone plates. A common factor is biocompatibility, but we will leave the studies and standards for pure materials or composite materials to the groups interested in materials. Design of plates has a major effect on performance. We have learned through clinical experience that plate application directly into the bone with loss of periosteum, either by stripping the periosteum or direct compression in the area of the undersurface of the plate, will cause loss of blood supply in the bone immediately under the plate and result in some bone necrosis immediately under the plate. This finding has, of course, caused a change in the design of plates, providing limited contact between the bone and the plate. Another factor entering into the picture is the stiffness of the plate. All bones to maintain strength and mineral content must be stressed continuously. Just simple immobilization in a splint will cause osteoporosis and weakening in a whole bone or bones not being used. Similarly, if we apply a stiff plate to bone, we will find that the bone is not stressed in the area of the plate, and osteopenia will occur. There is weakness of this area of bone compared to the area of bone exposed to ordinary stress from activity. Therefore, materials of various stiffness are being considered for use in bone plates.

The materials used for plates usually are nonabsorbable within the body. This means that after healing occurs, particularly with plates made of materials whose modulus of elasticity is more rigid than bone, the plate provides a stress riser at either end, and this creates the risk of fracture when sudden severe force is accidentally applied. Therefore, most plates, particularly in younger patients, are removed, thus necessitating a second operation with the risk of increased weakness at the site of empty screw holes for a period of time. Thus the possibility of bioresorbable plates has occurred. Factors to be considered in this instance are the initial strength of the bioresorbable plate and the rapidity of change in the strength of the plate as resorption takes place along with expected healing of the bone.

Hopefully the combination of weakening plate and strengthening bone will be maintained at or above normal strength through the healing period. We realize these are a few of the performance standards of concern. There are probably many more that we do not recognize as yet, but will become apparent as we follow our patients in the future.

This technical manual begins with Section I, entitled Screws, containing paper one, "The History and Development of Orthopedic Screws," by T. Sehlinger and D. Seligson. Although screw function in bone is a separate topic with separate standards, no discussion of plate performance can be done without recognition of the screw being part of the construct. We immediately realize that the screw design and its torque have an effect on a plate being held in place as discussed in paper two, "Effects of Design and Screw Torque on Stresses in Spinal and Fracture Plates: A Photoelastic Study," by A. Heiner and S. Brown.

Section II on Materials and Design deals with some of the basic portions of this subject. Paper three, by F. Baumgart and S. Perren entitled, "Rationale for the Design and Use of Pure Titanium for Internal Fixation Plates" and paper four by J. Disegi and D. Cesarone entitled "Metallurgical Properties of Unalloyed Titanium Limited Contact Dynamic Compression Plates," emphasize the difference in the modulus of elasticity between titanium and stainless steel (at present the most frequently used material to make plates). The less stiffness of the plate, the more opportunity for stress to pass through the bone while the plate is fixed to the bone. The concern about avascular necrosis under the plate is the reason for presenting paper five in this section, "The Concept of Biological Internal Fixation Using Limited Contact Plates," by F. Baumgart and S. Perren.

Section III, Testing Methods, contains those papers discussing testing methods. The first paper could be considered in Section II, since it discusses a new material for making plates polylactic acid. However, since the paper (number six), "Theoretical Strength Comparison of Bioresorbable (PLLA) Plates and Conventional Stainless Steel and Titanium Plates Used in Internal Fracture Fixation," by A. Nazre and S. Lin uses testing methods to compare the two plates, we have arbitrarily placed it in this section. This paper studied one of the bioresorbable plates now available, although it does not study change in strength as resorption occurs. It at least gives us a starting point and does discuss the first concern; does the plate have the strength to hold the bone in good position when first applied? The next paper (number seven), "Techniques in the Application of ISO 9585 Test Methods for the Determination of Bone

Plate Bending Properties," by D. Cesarone and J. Disegi compares the properties of stainless steel and titanium. It also discusses the limitations in performing the tests and the care needed to properly understand the values obtained. Paper eight, entitled "Cyclic Cantilever Fatigue Testing of Compression Hip Screw Plates," by R. Peterson, G. Lynch, and T. Brasher uses a simple mechanical bending test to make a comparison of the fatigue strength of the same area in different products.

Section IV, Clinical Application, has as a first paper (number nine), entitled "The Weakest Link in Bone-Plate-Fracture System; Changes with Time," by S. Kato, L. Latta, and T. Malinin presents an overview of our clinical problem in the application to maintain reduction of fractures and the weak sites occurring after the plate is removed. The second paper (number ten) in this section, entitled "Mechanical Evaluation of Internal and External Fixation for Metacarpal Fractures," by A. Ouellette, S. Kato, K. Nakamura, L. Latta, and W. Burkhalter compares the relative strength of types of fixation devices in a small bone, both freestanding and as contained in its normal anatomical setting. Another paper (number eleven), entitled "Biomechanics of Ulnar Osteotomies and Plate Fixation," by J. Rayhack, S. Glasser, E. Milne, and L. Latta compares the maintenance of reduction of an osteotomy site, which has been osteotomized (transected) in two different fashions. The last paper, number twelve in this publication, is a purely clinical paper demonstrating the end result of low contact dynamic compression plates in human beings. It is entitled "The 3.5 Millimeter Limited Contact Dynamic Compression Plate: A Preliminary Report of Technical Advantages," by J. Seiler, III, J. Jupiter, M. Miller, M. Albert, and M. Doxey.

This volume is not a definitive study, but rather provides us with a series of examples of our present status concerning the use of plates for the maintenance of reduction of fractures and factors pertaining to these plates. Using these studies and others in the literature, and more importantly, others to be conceived and performed, we hope to be able to better understand the clinical performance of bone plates and be able to write performance standards for this function.

To quote Dr. Ian Clark, a good friend and a long-time laborer on Committee F-4, "The two criteria of 'strength' and 'stiffness' will become increasingly important now that there are many advocates of titanium, plastic and composite plates, nails, and other fracture fixation systems. It is important that: (a) appropriate test methods be set up and (b) surgeons, manufacturers, and academic personnel have the same level of communication."

J. Paul Harvey Jr., M.D.
39 Congress St., Pasadena,
CA, 91105; symposium chairman
and editor.

Screws

Thomas E. Sehlinger,[1] and David Seligson[2]

HISTORY AND DEVELOPMENT OF THE ORTHOPEDIC SCREW

REFERENCE: Sehlinger, T. E., and Seligson, D., **"History and Development of the Orthopedic Screw,"** Clinical and Laboratory Performance of Bone Plates, ASTM STP 1217, J. P. Harvey, Jr. and R. F. Games, Eds., American Society for Testing and Materials, Philadelphia, 1994.

ABSTRACT: The orthopedic screw is the building block of internal fixation. Since screws were first used one hundred and fifty years ago for bone fixation, the concepts for their design have changed markedly. This paper reviews the milestones in the development of the orthopedic screw.

KEYWORDS: screw strength, screw diameter, core diameter, self-tapping

In 1850, M. Rigard of Strasbourg used one screw of unknown characteristics to secure a fracture of the olecranon, resulting in a "perfect cure" within two months. [1] By the turn of the century, Lane held that the screws were the most effective means to accurately oppose bone fragments to each other. [2]

In 1912, Sherman published an account of the desirable features of an orthopedic screw. [3] To decrease the risk of screw breakage, he recommended the use of screws with high ductility, such as those made from low carbon steel. He also suggested the screw head have a broad slit to allow the use of a broad screw driver and avoid slippage. He commended that screw heads be slightly rounded to add strength to the screw and allow for shallow countersinking. In addition, he suggested

---

[1]Resident, Department of Orthopedic Surgery, University of Louisville, Louisville, KY. 40292.

[2]Professor and Vice Chairman, Department of Orthopedic Surgery, University of Louisville, Louisville, KY. 40292.

that fully-threaded screws are the most efficient.
Sherman was one of many, including Lambotte and Hey-
Groves, who recommended using self-tapping machine screws
instead of tapered wood screws, since wood screw threads
do not bite the bone and are often manufactured of soft
steel [3,4,5] (Fig. 1). Sherman advocated using screws
with the composition of materials found in vanadium
screws, manufactured with .45 to .50 percent carbon, .70
to .90 percent magnesium, .09 to 1.10 percent chrome, .03
percent silicon, .18 percent vanadium, and the remaining
material iron. Lambotte, who was implanting screws in
Belgium during the time Sherman was practicing in the
United States, went a step further in screw technology by
developing machine-type screws especially designed for use
in bone. [4]

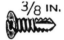

FIG. 1--Sherman's self-tapping machine screws

In the 1940's, Lyon and Peterson both found coarse
thread designs provided greater holding power in bone as
opposed to fine threads. While the thread design appears
to be the critical factor, Lyon noted the type of metal
employed in manufacturing the screw did have some effect
on holding power, as did the type of bone in which the
screw was inserted (cortical vs. cancellous). [6,7] it is
interesting to note that Lyon warned against applying too
much torque to a screw on insertion to avoid bone necrosis
around the threads and failure of the fixation device.
Peterson, after reviewing the types of orthopedic screws

used by the Army during World War II, found the
composition of metals employed that performs the best,
with regards to strength and inertness in the body, is the
steel 18-8 SMo, a high-alloy stainless steel containing 18
percent chromium, 8% nickel and 2% molybdenum.

Danis, in Théorie et Pratique de L'Ostéosynthèse,
proposed the use of screws that are adapted to the
characteristics of hard bone. [8] This work further
advanced the concept of screws designed for bone first
seen with Lambotte, who Danis had studied under years
before. Their implants were in contrast to the majority
of orthopedic screws in use at this time; screws that were
designed for metal and wood and adapted to use in bone.

Danis put forth three concepts in screw design
formulated from his years of experience with internal
fixation. First, the ratio of the exterior diameter to
core diameter should be three to two (metal screws are
typically four to three). Second, the surface of the
thread only needs be 1/6 of that for metal, bone is 1/6
the strength of metal. Third, the buttress thread design
should be utilized to provide the greatest holding power
in bone compared to the standard "V" thread of the day.
Although Danis had great success with internal fixation
utilizing these concepts of screw design, others had
difficulty duplicating his success rate (Fig. 2).

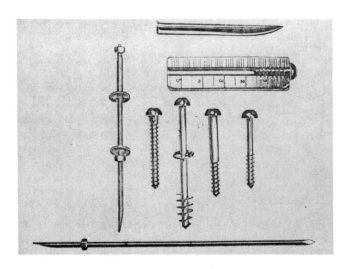

FIG. 2--Danis' specially designed bone screws

In the late 1950's, a group of surgeons and orthopedists met in Switzerland to discuss the poor success rate prevalent at that time in treatment of fractures with traction and plaster cast immobilization. Included in the group was M. Müller, a student of Danis. This meeting was the impetus for the formation of the ASIF (Association for the Study of Internal Fixation) or AO (Arbeitsgemeinschaft für Osteosynthesefragen) which enlisted Robert Mathys (a manufacturer) and Fritz Straumann (a metallurgist) to develop an armamentarium specifically for internal fixation. [9]   This instrumentation continued many of the concepts of screw design put forth by Danis.   The AO/ASIF group subsequently developed cortical and cancellous screws with buttress thread designs in common use today.   The cancellous screw was simply a lag screw, but as Schatzker noted, it would become the building block of internal fixation. [10]   The cortical screw can also be used as a lag screw by overdrilling the proximal cortex.

Bechtol further advanced screw design by suggesting a Phillips or Woodruff drive to reduce slippage during insertion.   He also found, as had Peterson, Lyon, and Danis, that coarse thread design is superior to the fine-threaded design in holding power, but questioned which provides the maximum strength against fatigue in-vivo.   In his studies, he found no advantage between self-tapping and non-self-tapping screws.   His major contribution, though, is experiments showing no bone necrosis when maximum torque was applied on the insertion of screws (a finding later supported by work done by the AO/ASIF). This was contradictory to the beliefs prior to his experiment, and contributed to the practice of fully tightening screws, thereby decreasing interfragmental motion. [11]

Screw strength studies, performed by Ansell and Scales in the late 1960's, found the weakest point in the orthopedic screw is the runout. [12]   In addition, their work shows, in contrast to Bechtol's, that pretapping screw holes allows for maximum holding power, and suggest using torque-limiting screw drivers to avoid exceeding the torsional yield strength of the screw.

In 1972, Hughes and Jordan showed the primary factor in screw strength is the core diameter of the screw.   They also showed the relative strengths of various popular materials used in screws, in terms of torque and tensile strength, proceeded in the order of En58J stainless steel> cast Co-Cr-Mo> titanium 160 (titanium alloy was found to be about equal to stainless steel).   The holding power of a screw was found to be independent of the screw's material, with the dependent factors shown to be the major diameter of the screw and shear strength of the bone. [13]

Danis' concept that the buttress-thread design provided the greatest holding power was disputed by the work of Koranyi, who showed no difference between the buttress and "V" thread design with regard to holding power. [14] Hughes and Jordan also suggested (and were later supported by Nunamaker and Perren) that the best screw head design to avoid slippage during insertion is a recessed hexagonal head. [15] Screws with this design were found to require three to four times less pressure for insertion.

The discussion of the best method of insertion, self-tapping versus non-self-tapping, continued with arguments supporting both sides. Finally, Schatzker showed that the manner of insertion as well as the thread design ("V" versus buttress) are minor factors in holding power of a screw in-vivo in an unloaded system. [16] His work supported that of Hughes and Jordan in that the primary characteristic of screw design affecting holding power is the screw diameter. This was elaborated upon further by Nunamaker and Perren citing the core diameter of a screw should be as large as conditions allow since the torque required to break a screw is largely determined by core diameter. [15]

Cannulated screws were developed from the same concept behind the Johansson cannulated Smith-Petersen hip nail, i.e., improved precision of insertion. Cannulated screws were not widely used, however, since it was difficult to control wall thickness and hence strength. Since 1985, automated manufacturing methods with laser-guided gun drills improved precision so that bone screws with a favorable wall-to-cannulation ratio can be fabricated. The dimension of these screws were designed to provide a minor diameter greater than the minor diameter of the corresponding uncannulated screws. Thus a large cannulated screw has a minor diameter of 4.5mm which is greater than the 3.2mm diameter of the corresponding large cancellous bone screw. Experiments using screws of various designs and composition over the last twenty years have shown the most important parameter, in screw strength and holding power, is the screw diameter. Cannulated screws have been shown to have significantly increased strength, in terms of bending, tension, and torsion, when compared to cancellous screws with the same major diameter. [17] The biomechanical parameters of the cannulated screw are presently being investigated, but early experiments seem to indicate the cannulated screw will be at least equal to, if not greater, in terms of holding power, to the corresponding-sized cancellous and cortical screws. [17] This, coupled with the greater precision and control seen with the cannulated screws secondary to placement over guide pins, could increase the overall usage of these screws. (Fig. 3).

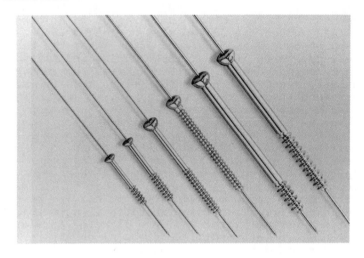

FIG. 3--A family of cannulated screws (courtesy of Johnson and Johnson, New Brunswick, New Jersey [18]

Today new materials including absorbables are being introduced into clinical practice. Computer-assisted manufacturing allows the fabrication of more specialized screws such as tapered screws for spinal pedicle fixation and screws with variable pitch. Doubtless more advances will occur in the orthopedic screw by the turn of the century then took place in the past one hundred and fifty years.

CONCLUSION

The orthopedic screw has evolved over the years, encompassing a variety of shapes, designs, and compositions. Advances in technology have allowed corresponding advances in the biomechanical features of the bone screw to include those features which provide the greatest stability _in-vivo_. As orthopedic surgery advances, hopefully it will continue to take advantage of the continuing developments in bone screw design.

REFERENCES

[1]   Rigaud, M., "Des Vis Metalliques Enfoncées Dans Le Tissu des Os, pour le traîtement de certaines fractures," _Revue Medico Chirurgicale De Paris_, Vol. 8, 1850, p 113.

[2] Lane, W., "The Operative Treatment of Simple Fractures," Surgery, Gynecology and Obstetrics, Vol. 8, 1909, pp 344-354.

[3] Sherman, W., "Vanadium Steel Bone Plates and Screws," Surgery, Gynecology and Obstetrics, Vol. 14, 1912, pp 629-634.

[4] Lambotte, A., Chirurgie Opératoire Des Fractures, Mason and Cie, Paris, 1913, p 52.

[5] Hey-Groves, E., On Modern Methods of Treating Fractures, William Wood and Co., New York, 1916, pp 201-202.

[6] Lyon, W., "Actual Holding Power of Various Screws in Bone," Annals of Surgery, Vol. 3, 1941, pp 376-384.

[7] Peterson, L., "Fixation of Bones by Plates and Screws," Journal of Bone and Joint Surgery, Vol. 29, 1947, pp 335-347.

[8] Danis, R., Théorie et Pratique de L'Ostéosynthèse, Paris Libraries de L'Academie de Medecine, 1949, pp 75-86.

[9] Allgower, M., "Internal Fixations of Fractures: Evolution of Concepts," Clinical Orthopedics, Vol. 138, 1979, pp 26-29.

[10] Schatzker, J., "Principles of Stable Internal Fixation," Canadian Journal of Surgery, Vol. 23, 1980, pp 232-235.

[11] Bechtol, C., Metals and Engineering in Bone and Joint Surgery, Williams and Wilken Co., Baltimore, 1959, pp 107-166.

[12] Ansell, R. and Scales, J., "A study of Some Factors which Affect the Strength of Screws and Their Insertion and Holding Power in Bone," Journal of Biomechanics, Vol. 1, 1968, pp 279-302.

[13] Hughes, A. N. and Jordan, B.A., "The Mechanical Properties of Surgical Bone Screws and some Aspects of Insertion Practice," Injury, Vol. 4, 1972, p 25.

[14] Koranyi, E., "Holding Power of Orthopedic Screws in Bone," Clinical Orthopedics, Vol. 72, 1970, pp 283-302.

[15] Nunamaker, D. and Perren, S., "Force Measurement in Screw Fixation," Journal of Biomechanics, Vol. 9, 1976, p 669.

Anneliese D. Heiner,[1] and Stanley A. Brown[1]

EFFECTS OF DESIGN AND SCREW TORQUE ON STRESSES IN SPINAL AND FRACTURE
FIXATION PLATES: A PHOTOELASTIC STUDY

REFERENCE: Heiner, A. D., and Brown, S. A., "Effects of Design and
Screw Torque on Stresses in Spinal and Fracture Fixation Plates: A
Photoelastic Study," Clinical and Laboratory Performance of Bone
Plates, ASTM STP 1217, J. P. Harvey, Jr. and R. F. Games, Eds.,
American Society for Testing and Materials, Philadelphia, 1994.

ABSTRACT: The stresses on an orthopaedic device are dependent on the
dimensional design of the device and the applied loads. The stresses on
spinal plates and fracture fixation plates were studied using
photoelastic stress analysis. Photoelastic spinal plate models revealed
the areas of stress concentration and the expansion behavior of the
plates, when a screw was screwed down into a plate slot. Photoelastic
fracture fixation plate models attached to bone models showed relative
stresses as the amount of bending, screw tightness, plate width, and
hole spacing were varied. This photoelastic study and others like it
can evaluate potential designs or design changes for orthopaedic
devices.

KEYWORDS: device design, fracture fixation plates, photoelastic stress
analysis, polymer composites, spinal plates, stress concentrations

---

There is a wide variety of orthopaedic devices, representing both
design improvements and devices for different applications. A paper
published in 1956 pointed to the need to study internal fixation and
prosthetic devices from an engineering point of view [1]. The author
recognized that studies were needed on the design and fabrication of
orthopaedic devices, in addition to the earlier studies on the metals
used and the body's reaction to them. A more recent impetus for
studying design and fabrication of orthopaedic devices is the
availability of alternative materials such as carbon fiber reinforced
polymer composites. Considerable variations in fiber reinforcement and
processing techniques are possible for polymer composites. These
variations affect the mechanical properties of the polymer composite.
In turn, these variations may either limit or allow more freedom in

---

[1]Graduate student and Associate professor, respectively,
Department of Biomedical Engineering, Case Western Reserve University,
Cleveland, OH 44106.

considering other design issues for orthopaedic devices.

One technique that can indicate areas or dimensions to redesign is photoelastic stress analysis [2,3]. Photoelastic stress analysis determines the stress distribution and stress concentrations on a part. Photoelastic techniques have been used previously to study the stresses on bones with fracture fixation plates [1,4,5]. When compared to other techniques of stress analysis, photoelastic stress analysis is quick, simple and accurate. It is especially suited for evaluating the effects of a notch, hole or other discontinuity on the piece. Orthopaedic devices and the bones to which they are attached contain holes; photoelastic stress analysis can help determine the effects of these holes.

Two types of orthopaedic devices were studied using photoelasticity: spinal plates and fracture fixation plates. The spinal plates used were part of the variable screw placement (VSP) system developed in 1982 for use in posterior lumbar interbody fusion [6-8]. The fracture fixation plates used were modelled after a 4.5 mm, round-hole, normal fracture fixation plate. The stiffness and fracture strength of different fracture fixation plate designs have been compared [9-15]. The purpose of this study was to use photoelastic techniques to study the effects of design and screw torque on these orthopaedic devices.

PROCEDURE

Models of spinal plates and fracture fixation plates were machined from photoelastic material (MicroMeasurements, Inc.). The models were stressed, then viewed between crossed polarizing filters. The colors, or fringe orders, which are seen at each point are directly proportional to the difference in the principal stresses at that point [2]. The fringe pattern on the entire piece shows the points of high stress. These points, called stress concentrations, can help indicate design changes. Fringe orders at free boundaries such as edges or holes are directly proportional to the stresses at those points, and can be used to compare stresses between different free boundaries.

Spinal Plates

Spinal plates made out of photoelastic material were used to analyze stresses and study expansion behavior as transpedicular screw nuts were screwed down into the plate slots. Variables studied were screw position and screw tightness. A transpedicular screw nut was screwed down into a spinal plate slot at one of two positions: at the outer edge of a slot (edge position), or at the center of a slot (center position), as shown in Fig. 1. Screw tightness was measured with a torque wrench (GSE Inc., Model 1125-50). The plates were photographed between crossed polarizing filters after application of incremental increases of torque, to study the fringe patterns. In a separate experiment, after application of incremental increases in torque, the width of the photoelastic spinal plates was measured with a micrometer at three locations: at the center bridge, and at the center of each of

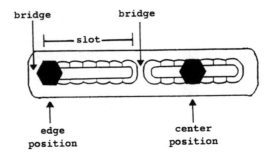

FIG. 1--Terminology for regions on a spinal plate.

the two slots (Fig. 1). Percent expansion was calculated at each
location for each incremental increase in torque.

Fracture Fixation Plates

The photoelastic study of fracture fixation plates involved
placing different photoelastic plate designs under some of the types of
loads anticipated in the service of a fracture fixation plate. The
loads were from tightening screws, or from 4-point bending.

The plate models were machined from 6.35 mm (1/4 in.) thick
photoelastic material. Dimensions for the plate models came from a 4.5
mm, eight-hole, normal fracture fixation plate. The bone models were
machined from 6.35 mm (1/4 in.) thick plexiglass, with hole spacings
matching the hole spacings for the plate models, and a transverse break
at the middle of the piece. The screws used for the bone/plate assembly
were 4.5 mm cortical bone screws.

The plates were attached to the fractured bone models with the
cortical bone screws. All screws were tightened to the same torque in a
given experiment with a torque wrench (GSE Inc., Model 1125-50). The
bone/plate assembly was then placed into a 4-point bending device, with
the plate model on the tension side. Bending loads of different
magnitudes were applied to the bone/plate assembly. At each bending
load, the bone/plate assembly was viewed between crossed polarizing
filters. The fringe orders at the hole boundaries were recorded and
analyzed. Comparison of different model designs indicated the effects
of design and screw torque.

Variations in screw tightness, plate width, and hole spacing of
photoelastic plate models patterned after the fracture fixation plate
were studied (Table 1). Varying the amount of screw tightness (the
torque applied to the fixating screws) allowed for viewing the
development of the stress patterns with increasing fixation. Varying
plate width and hole spacing were two design changes possible for
fracture fixation plates. The effect of hole position along the plate
was also studied.

TABLE 1--*Variations in screw tightness, plate width,*
and hole spacing of photoelastic plate models.

	Screw Tightness, N·m	Plate Width, mm	Hole Spacing, mm
Vary screw tightness	0.05	19	16
	0.07	19	16
	0.10	19	16
Vary plate width	0.05	11	16
	0.05	13	16
	0.05	16	16
	0.05	19	16
Vary hole spacing	0.05	16	13
	0.05	16	16
	0.05	16	19

The original plate had width = 11 mm and hole spacing = 16 mm.

Fringe orders were measured at the hole edges, along the minimum cross-sections of the plate. Each of the eight holes then had two points where a fringe order was measured. The fringe orders that were measured were divided into four positions, each position consisting of four points which should be equivalent by symmetry. For instance, the outermost position consisted of the two points at the outermost hole at one end of the piece, plus the two points at the outermost hole at the other end of the piece. Fringe orders were also measured at the hole edges, between the holes, along the long axis of the plate. These fringe orders were measured when only screw tightness was applied.

One way to compare designs is to plot fringe order versus applied load [2]. The best design gives the smallest slope, since that design develops the least stress as applied load is increased. The y-intercept represented an additional parameter; namely, the stress on the plate model resulting from just screw tightness. For this study, both slopes and y-intercepts from these plots were compared. The fringe orders at the hole edges, between the holes, along the long axis of the plate, when only screw torque was applied, were also studied.

To calculate slope and y-intercept, the measured fringe orders were first averaged for each position. Slope and y-intercept values were then calculated across the bending loads, at each position. The number of trials was 5, except for when studying the effects of higher screw tightness, where the number of trials was 3. Whether or not the slopes and y-intercepts were significantly different was determined using ANOVA and Duncan's multiple range test [16]. The level of significance was $\alpha = 0.01$ except where otherwise stated.

a)

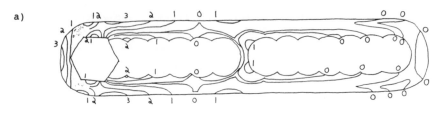

b)

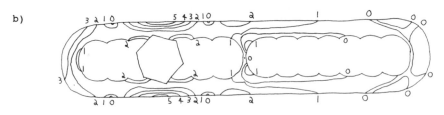

FIG. 2--Fringe patterns of photoelastic spinal plates under screw torque
applied at the (a) edge and (b) center position. For the edge position,
the applied torque was 0.20 N·m. For the center position, the applied
torque was 0.10 N·m. Numbers indicate fringe orders; high numbers
indicate stress concentrations.

RESULTS

Spinal Plates

The highest fringe orders, indicating the highest stresses, were
located around the transpedicular screw nut (Fig. 2). The center
position developed higher stresses than did the edge position. The
fringe patterns extended to the opposite side of the spinal plate.

For both the edge and center positions, the spinal plates expanded
in a seesaw manner; the width of one side went up, the width of the
other side went down, and the middle stayed constant (Fig. 3). With
increasing screw torque, the slot with the nut being screwed down
expanded, and the other slot contracted. The width of the center bridge
did not change significantly. There was more expansion (and
contraction) when the nut was in the center position, than when the nut
was in the edge position.

Fracture Fixation Plates

As screw tightness increased, there was no significant difference
between the slopes, at the two outermost positions. There was
significant difference between the slopes, at the innermost position (α
= 0.01) and at the second innermost position (α = 0.05). The y-
intercept at all positions and the fringe orders between the holes
increased significantly as screw tightness increased, and the increases
were linear ($r^2 \geq 0.972$) (Fig. 4).

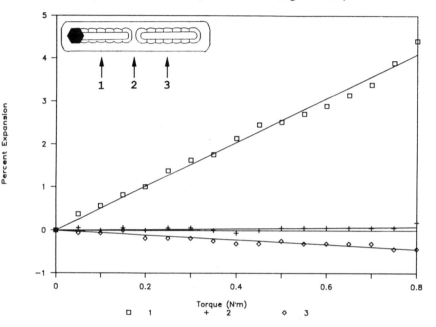

Spinal Plate Expansion, Edge Torque

FIG. 3--Expansion behavior of a photoelastic spinal plate under screw torque applied at the edge position. The expansion behavior was like a seesaw, with the center bridge acting as a pivot point.

In general, as plate width increased, slope and y-intercept decreased, although not always significantly (Fig. 5). At the outermost hole position, the slopes for the four plate widths studied were not significantly different. At the innermost hole position, the slopes for the four plate widths studied were all significantly different. As the hole spacing increased, there was no significant difference between the slopes at the innermost hole position.

The slope increased significantly as the hole position got closer to the center; this result was consistent across changes in screw tightness, plate width, and hole spacing (Fig. 6). The slope for the outermost position was much lower than the slopes for the other positions; this slope was significantly lower than for the other positions, in all but one case. The y-intercept for the outermost position was significantly higher than the y-intercept for the other positions, in all but two cases (and in all but one case at $\alpha = 0.05$).

The fringe orders measured between the holes were higher than the fringe orders measured at the minimum cross-sections of the piece, when only screw torque was applied.

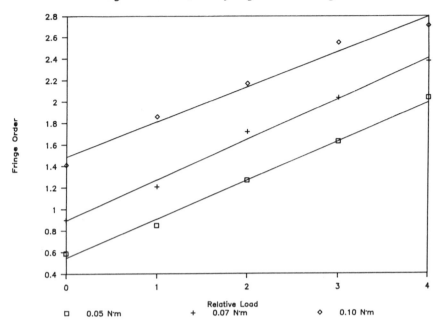

FIG. 4--Effects of varying screw tightness on plate stress. The stress
due to screw tightness (y-intercept) increased linearly with increasing
screw tightness. This plate had width = 19 mm, and hole spacing = 16
mm; the hole position was the second innermost position.

DISCUSSION

Spinal Plates

     The photoelastic spinal plates showed that stress concentrations
occurred around the transpedicular screw nut. The plates also showed
that the center position developed higher stresses than did the edge
position. These results were consistent with the results from an
earlier experiment, in which polymer composite spinal plates were tested
to failure using the same procedure as for the photoelastic spinal
plates. Areas indicated as stress concentrations on the photoelastic
plates corresponded with the areas of fracture on the polymer composite
spinal plates. The photoelastic plates showed that the center position
was more highly stressed than the edge position; for the polymer
composite spinal plates, the center position failed at lower screw
torques than did the edge position. The stress on the center position
could be reduced by decreasing each slot length or increasing the plate
width. However, decreasing the slot length would reduce the ability to
choose a screw location which comes with a larger slot length.
Increasing the plate width must be balanced by the anatomical space

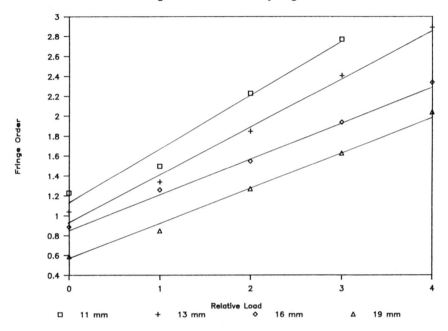

FIG. 5--Effects of varying plate width on plate stress. As the width
increased, the stresses due to both screw tightness (y-intercept) and
bending loads (slope) decreased. This plate had hole spacing = 16 mm,
and screw tightness = 0.05 N·m; the hole position was the second
innermost position.

available and the dangers of stress protection by a plate which is too
wide and strong. Polymer composites, which can produce less stress
protection than metals, may allow for increasing the width without
increasing the risk of stress protection.

Expansion behavior from one screw in a plate slot might be offset
by the expansion behavior from a screw in the other plate slot. The
stress patterns extended to the opposite side of the spinal plate, where
they would combine with stress patterns produced by another screw.
Although the width of the center bridge did not change significantly
over the range of torques studied, the stress on the center bridge
increased, as indicated by photoelastic stress analysis. The center
bridge was also one of the fracture sites for the polymer composite
spinal plates, further indicating that this area had an increased amount
of stress.

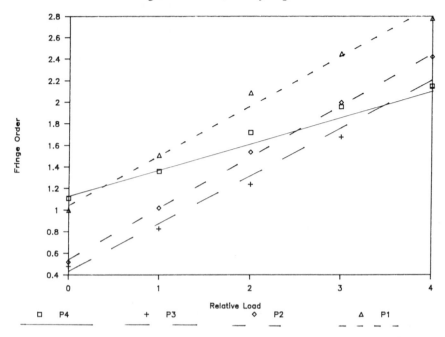

Fringe Orders, Varying Position

FIG. 6--Effects of the position along the plate on plate stress. Hole positions are designated as P1 through P4, with P1 representing the innermost holes and P4 representing the outermost holes. At the outermost hole position (P4), the stress due to bending loads (slope) was significantly lower than at the other positions, and the stress due to screw tightness (y-intercept) was significantly higher than at the other positions. This plate had width = 16 mm, hole spacing = 13 mm, and screw tightness = 0.05 N·m.

Fracture Fixation Plates

As screw tightness increased, there was no significant difference in the stress due to bending (slope) at the two outermost positions. However, the stress due to bending was significantly different at the two innermost positions. This indicated that the increase in stress on the plate, as a bending load was applied, was independent of the screw tightness at the two outermost positions, but dependent on the screw tightness at the two innermost positions. The stresses due to bending at the outermost positions were not affected by screw tightness. The innermost positions, being closer to the bone fracture site, had a more complicated stress state, which was affected by the screw tightness.

As screw tightness increased, the stress due to screw tightness (y-intercept) increased significantly over the range studied, and the increases were linear. This could indicate a linear relationship between screw tightness and plate stress in actual fracture fixation plates.

An increase in plate width decreased the stresses due to screw tightness (y-intercept), and the stresses due to bending (slope). In practice, the strongest piece is the one with the smallest hole [2]. As plate width increased, the size of the screw hole, relative to the plate width, decreased, resulting in a relatively stronger plate. The width of the plate affected the stress due to bending at the innermost holes, but did not affect the stress due to bending at the outermost holes. This suggests use of a tapered-width plate, where the width of the plate decreases from the innermost holes to the outermost holes, similar to a tapered-width plate proposed previously [17].

When the hole spacing was varied, the stress due to bending (slope) did not change significantly at the innermost holes. This was consistent with a previous study which found that increasing the hole spacing did not change the tension on the screws in the innermost holes [9]. The innermost screw holes experience the greatest stress when a plate is first applied to a fractured bone [9,15,18,19]. Previous studies indicate that the longer a fracture fixation plate, the better [11,14]. Increasing the hole spacing is one way to increase the length of the plate, without affecting the stress on the innermost holes. This might be a better way to increase plate length than by increasing the number of screws [15].

The position farthest away from the fracture had the smallest increase in stress due to bending (slope), in all but one case studied. Single-cortex screws are sometimes used in the outermost holes of a fracture fixation plate [20]. Single-cortex screws give less strength to the fixation of the plate to bone than do double-cortex screws. Although the strength of fixation is less, the stress on the plate is also less, so this lesser stress can be tolerated.

The position farthest away from the fracture had the largest stress due to screw tightness (y-intercept), in nearly all of the cases studied. This meant that the outermost holes were the most highly stressed when no bending was applied. The outermost holes, being closest to the edges of the piece, had less material around them, and thus carried more stress.

When a plate model was first screwed down onto a bone model, the highest stress occurred between the holes rather than at a minimum cross-section between a hole and an edge of the plate. This indicated that when a plate is first screwed down, plate failure may preferentially occur between the holes. This has occurred with a polymer composite fracture fixation plate, in conjunction with a processing weakness [21].

There are many other dimensional variations that could be investigated for fracture fixation plates. Possibilities include changing hole spacing while keeping length constant, changing length while keeping hole spacing constant, changing the thickness, and using two rows of screws instead of one. Other experimental variations include the type of fracture, applied load, and degree of bone healing. Oblique, spiral and comminuted fractures are more common than the transverse fracture studied here [22]. Loads such as other bending directions, tension, compression, and torsion could be studied. Photoelastic stress analysis of the stresses seen on a plate attached to a healed bone could also be done.

More complex experimental setups can be used for studying other orthopaedic design applications. For instance, using a photoelastic coating on a piece, instead of using bulk photoelastic material, would show changes in stress on the piece due to transverse bending, and would be useful for more complicated shapes. The orthopaedic device could be attached to an actual bone or to a bone model with a more realistic shape than the one used here.

CONCLUSION

Photoelastic stress analysis is a design technique which can be applied to orthopaedic devices. This study used a relatively simple setup which generated data for comparative purposes, and gave results consistent with earlier studies.

For spinal plates, photoelastic stress analysis showed areas which were stress concentrations, and showed which screw position was more highly stressed. These results were confirmed by polymer composite spinal plates tested in a similar manner. Expansion behavior of photoelastic spinal plates resembled a seesaw; as screw torque increased, the width of one side went up, and the width of the other side went down.

For fracture fixation plates attached to bone models, photoelastic stress analysis showed how stresses changed with variations in screw tightness, amount of bending, plate width, and hole spacing. There was a linear relationship between screw tightness and the stress due to the screw tightness. The increase in stress due to bending was independent of the screw tightness at the two outermost hole positions, but not at the two innermost hole positions. The stresses on the plate models decreased as plate width increased. The increase in stress due to bending was independent of hole spacing, at the innermost holes. The outermost holes developed the least stress from the bending loads, and the most stress from the screw tightness alone.

ACKNOWLEDGEMENTS

This study was supported in part by NIH Training Grant 5-T32-GM07535, the W.O. Frohring Foundation, and the National Science Foundation. The authors wish to thank the Cleveland Clinic Foundation for equipment and technical assistance.

REFERENCES

[1] Martz, C.D., "Stress Tolerance of Bone and Metal," _Journal of Bone and Joint Surgery_, Vol. 38A, No. 4, 1956, pp 827-834.

[2] Heywood, R.B., _Designing by Photoelasticity_, Chapman & Hall Ltd., London, 1952.

[3] Tech Note TN-702-1: "Introduction to Stress Analysis by the PhotoStress Method," Measurements Group, Inc., Raleigh, NC, 1989.

[4] Rybicki, E.F., etal, "Mathematical and Experimental Studies on the Mechanics of Plated Transverse Fractures," _Journal of Biomechanics_, Vol. 7, 1974, pp 377-384.

[5] Shelton, J.C., Gorman, D., and Bonfield, W., "The Application of Holography to Examine Plated Fracture Fixation Systems," _Journal of Materials Science: Materials in Medicine_, Vol. 1, 1990, pp 146-153.

[6] Steffee, A.D., "The Variable Screw Placement System with Posterior Lumbar Interbody Fusion," _Lumbar Interbody Fusion: Principles and Techniques in Spine Surgery_, P. M. Lin and K. Gill, Eds., Aspen Publishers, Inc., Rockville, MD, 1989, pp 81-93.

[7] Steffee, A.D., Biscup, R.S., and Sitkowski, D.J., "Segmental Spine Plates with Pedicle Screw Fixation: A New Internal Fixation Device for Disorders of the Lumbar and Thoracolumbar Spine," _Clinical Orthopaedics and Related Research_, Vol. 203, 1986, pp 45-53.

[8] Wenz, L.M., Brown, S.A., Moet, A., Merritt, K., and Steffee, A., "Accelerated Testing of a Composite Spine Plate," _Composites_, Vol. 20, No. 6, 1989, pp 569-574.

[9] Laurence, M., Freeman, M.A.R., and Swanson, S.A.V., "Engineering Considerations in the Internal Fixation of Fractures of the Tibial Shaft," _Journal of Bone and Joint Surgery_, Vol. 51B, No. 4, 1969, pp 754-768.

[10] Laurence, M., Freeman, M.A.R., and Swanson, S.A.V., "The Internal Fixation of Long Bone Shaft Fractures: Engineering Considerations," _Proceedings of the Royal Society of Medicine_, Vol. 59, 1966, p 943.

[11] Levine, D.L., and Stoneking, J.E., "A Three Dimensional, Finite Element Based, Parametric Study of an Orthopaedic Bone Plate _In Situ_," _International Conference on Finite Elements in Biomechanics_, February 18-20, 1980, Tucson, AZ, pp 713-728.

[12] Lindahl, O., "The Rigidity of Fracture Immobilization with Plates," _Acta Orthopaedica Scandinavica_, Vol. 38, 1967, pp 101-114.

[13] Lindahl, O., "Rigidity of Immobilization of Transverse Fractures," _Acta Orthopaedica Scandinavica_, Vol. 32, 1962, pp 237-246.

[14] Ray, D.R., Ledbetter, W.B., Bynum, D., and Boyd, C.L., "A Parametric Analysis of Bone Fixation Plates on Fractured Equine Third Metacarpal," _Journal of Biomechanics_, Vol. 4, 1971, pp 163-174.

[15] Sherman, W.O., "Vanadium Steel Bone Plates and Screws," _Surgery, Gynecology and Obstetrics_, Vol. 14, 1912, pp 629-634.

[16] Dougherty, E.R., _Probability and Statistics for the Engineering, Computing, and Physical Sciences_, Prentice-Hall, Inc., Englewood Cliffs, NJ, 1990.

[17] Frankel, V.H., and Burstein, A.H., _Orthopaedic Biomechanics: The Application of Engineering to the Musculoskeletal System_, Lea &

Febiger, Philadelphia, 1970.

[18]   Cheal, E.J., Hays, W.C., and White, A.A., "Stress Analysis of a Simplified Compression Plate Fixation System for Fractured Bones," Computers and Structures, Vol. 17, No. 5-6, 1983, pp 845-855.

[19]   Szivek, J.A., "A Testing Technique Allowing Cyclic Application of Axial, Bending, and Torque Loads to Fracture Plates to Examine Screw Loosening," Journal of Biomedical Materials Research, Vol. 21, No. A3, April 1989, pp 105-116.

[20]   Muller, M.E., Allgower, M., and Willenegger, H., Manual of Internal Fixation, Springer-Verlag, Berlin, 1970.

[21]   Gillett, N., Brown, S.A., Dumbleton, J.H., and Pool, R.P., "The Use of Short Carbon Fibre Reinforced Thermoplastic Plates for Fracture Fixation," Biomaterials, Vol. 6, 1985, pp 113-121.

[22]   Rybicki, E.F., and Simonen, F.A., "Mechanics of Oblique Fracture Fixation Using a Finite-Element Model," Journal of Biomechanics, Vol. 10, 1977, pp 141-148.

Materials & Design

Frank W. Baumgart,[1] and Stephan M. Perren[2]

RATIONALE FOR THE DESIGN AND USE OF PURE TITANIUM INTERNAL FIXATION PLATES

REFERENCE: Baumgart, F. W., and Perren, S. M., "Rationale for the Design and use of Pure Titanium Internal Fixation Plates," Clinical and Laboratory Performance of Bone Plates, ASTM STP 1217, J. P. Harvey, Jr., and R. F. Games, Eds., American Society for Testing and Materials, Philadelphia, 1994.

ABSTRACT: Commercially pure titanium is standardized by ISO 5832-2 and has better fatigue strength than stainless steel. Its other mechanical properties are comparable to the properties of stainless steel. Bone plates need contouring in most cases of application. A retrospective evaluation of more than 500 clinical cases showed that the initiated strain by contouring is on average about 1.6% below the elongation at fracture for cp titanium. Therefore, contouring of titanium plates having equivalent design to stainless steel plates is not critical.
The most important properties of pure titanium are its excellent biocompatibility and its corrosion resistance. The metal is protected by a very thin and tough layer of titanium oxide. Anodizing gives the titanium oxide layer a certain color.
No allergic reactions to cp titanium are known so far. The debris of titanium caused by relative movement of implant parts which are in contact consists of titanium oxide and has a dark color. This may be sometimes undesirable for cosmetic reasons but the particles do not contain any toxic element.

Pure Titanium is an appropriate material for bone plates and screws used for internal fixation.

KEYWORDS: pure titanium, bone plate, contouring, toxicity, allergy, strain, bending, handling, elongation .

[1] Head of AOTK Product Information, Clavadelerstr., CH-7270 Davos Platz, Switzerland

[2] Head of AO Research Institute, Clavadelerstr., CH-7270 Davos Platz, Switzerland

MECHANICAL REQUIREMENTS FOR MATERIALS FOR BONE PLATES

Introduction

Standardized metallic materials for internal fixation implants
are stainless steel and titanium. Stainless steel was used first as an
implant material at the beginning of this century (Lane 1914, [1],
Lambotte 1913, [2]). Titanium has been used for more than 30 years for
implants (Beder and Eade, 1956, [3]). The majority of internal
fixation implants are still made from stainless steel, but the
application of titanium implants is increasing.

Strength and stiffness

Bone plates have to perform a certain biomechanical function: To
build a sufficiently stable and stiff structure to withstand, together
with the bone, functional load. Metals with high strength and
stiffness allow for designing of implants with small dimensions which
is a general advantage for any implant, also for plates.

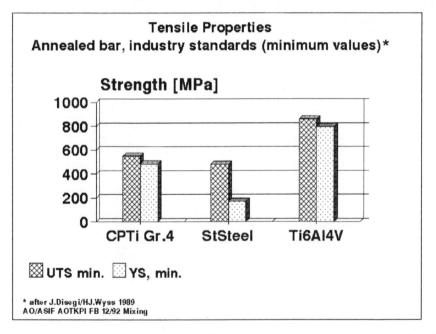

FIG.1--Mechanical properties of implant materials for internal fixation
(minimum values for annealed materials)

Plate contouring

Plates for internal fixation of bone fractures have to be
contoured for anatomically different locations. This is of less
importance for the diaphyses of long bones than for the proximal and

distal parts of these bones. Also the special geometries of the pelvis or of the spine show a much more prominent curvature of the bone surface requiring adaptation of the plate.

The majority of the straight plates need a more or less special adaptation ("contouring") by the surgeon to perform well in fracture fixation. Therefore, a certain amount of ductility of such plates is desirable. In other words: The plate material should have a sufficient elongation at fracture.

Appropriate instrumentation for safe contouring is necessary.

Frankle et al.,[4] showed in a retrospective study of X-rays based on 500 documented cases of tibial fractures that the applied strain for contouring of straight plates is between 0.6 and 16% with an average of 1.6 %. The currently used plate materials stainless steel and titanium show elongation at fracture of more than 12%, which is sufficiently safe in the case of closely contoured plates (see Plate contouring of stainless steel plates).

It is also evident that a uniform strength of a plate helps to avoid sharp curvatures in bending or twisting of the plate.

If we substitute a stainless steel implant by a cp titanium version we have to increase slightly the dimensions if we require the same failure load. The long-term experience with stainless steel implants is a good basis for designing titanium implants for similar or identical applications.

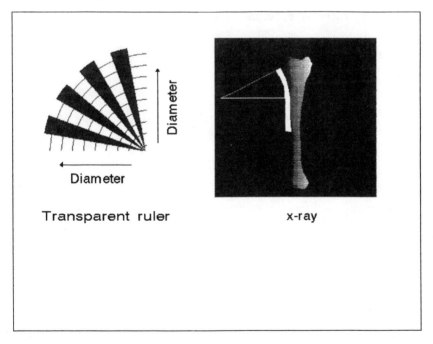

Transparent ruler   **x-ray**

FIG.2--The method of Frankle for determination of plate curvatures in clinical cases.

    The mechanical properties of stainless steel are excellent,
pure titanium does not reach completely the strength and elongation
(Fig.1) of this "old" material. However, the fatigue strength of
titanium is better than that of steel and the modulus of elasticity
(the material stiffness) and the density are less, which may have
certain advantages. The costs of titanium per kg are somewhat higher
than those of stainless steel. The resistance of titanium against
repeated plastic deformation is less than that of stainless steel.
Therefore, the repeated bending of plates should be avoided at all
costs (This is also true for stainless steel plates).

Titanium alloys

    The mechanical strength of the titanium alloys used for surgical
implants is generally about 10 to 20% higher than that of cp titanium.
    Steinemann discussed recently the status of titanium and its
alloys [5]. The paper favours the beta alloy Ti15Mo5Zr3Al which has
higher strength and elongation at fracture. Experience regarding
application and biocompatibility of this new alloy is still limited.
It is not commercially available yet. The future will show the
importance of this new material.
    Recently, the titanium aluminum niobium alloy Ti6Al7Nb [6] seems
to be the appropriate solution if higher strength is required.

THE BIOCOMPATIBILITY OF TITANIUM

Standards

    The most important advantage of pure titanium is its
biocompatibility. It is well accepted and proven. An ISO standard (ISO
5832-2) exists for cp titanium [7]. Clinical experience exists for
titanium implants of more than 30 years of application [8],[3].
    Titanium alloys (Ti6Al4V [9], Ti6Al7Nb [10] and Ti5Al2.5Fe [11])
are also standardized or are waited to be standardized soon. They are
accepted worldwide as biomaterials with an acceptable risk.

Surface treatment

    Anodizing--To avoid "mixing" of stainless steel and titanium
implants, the titanium implants (of the AO/ASIF) get a surface
treatment which gives them a golden color caused by an optical effect.
    A very thin titanium oxide layer (a few Angstroms thick) is
generated by an anodizing process and selects certain frequencies of
the visible light. Furthermore, the anodized layer protects the device
better against abrasive attack than a non-anodized surface.
    Anodizing does not change the biocompatibility of the device
because titanium is always stabilized by a titanium oxide layer. The
anodized surface simply shows a different homogenized organization of
this layer [12].

Roughness--It might be that the adhesion and the type of the living tissue at the metal surface depends upon the geometrical structure (e.g. roughness of the surface) rather than the material itself. Such observations have been made by investigators of porous structures on hip joint prostheses, where certain pore sizes and porosities showed different adaptation of the tissue to the surface structure. Cell sizes in comparison to local characteristic surface dimensions probably play a role independent of the chemical and metallurgical properties of the material.

Toxicity

Gerber and Perren [13] have proven the biocompatibility of Titanium in toxicity tests using embryonic rat femora. There are no toxic effects known from pure titanium.

The most common titanium alloy, the Ti6A14V contains 4% vanadium. Vanadium has been shown to be a toxic metal. But the behavior when used as part of an alloy is different from the behavior of the pure metal. The solubility (degradation) of this and similar extremely corrosion resistant alloys is negligible and the low content of toxic substances also prevents a remarkable emission of toxic ions from the metal surface under normal circumstances. In the case of substantial wear, the situation may change.

However, if the existence of a toxic element in an alloy can be avoided this alternative solution should be preferred. Therefore, the use of pure titanium or of titanium alloys (e.g. Ti6A17Nb) without toxic elements is preferable for implants for internal fixation.

Allergy

S. Hierholzer [14] reported extensive investigations on patients with metal implants and showed an increase of allergic reactions to metallic implants during the last 20 years.

Commercially pure titanium is a material which has shown until today no adverse effects to the human body. Allergic reactions to pure titanium have not been observed so far. The investigations of Hierholzer confirmed that the number of complications in the case of allergic patients with metal implants was significantly higher than in the case of non-allergic patients with implants. The authors recommend titanium for use in patients who may have metal allergy.

Wear

Most of the implants used for internal fixation are not intended to function under conditions of relative motion (like an artificial joint). Therefore, wear resistance is not a priority aspect. However, in the case of unstable osteosyntheses, there might be a local sliding between the plate hole surface and screwhead. This motion creates wear particles. Regarding these particles we have to consider that:
    1. The stainless steel particles contain toxic nickel and chromium ions and may show brown or black color in case of reported metallosis [14].
    2. The titanium particles are dark colored and contain titanium oxide.

The dark color of titanium oxide sometimes may not be desired for cosmetic reasons especially in case of thin soft tissue cover. However, titanium oxide is proven to be biologically inert and extremely tissue friendly.

Electrochemical behavior

Steinemann [15] stated that titanium cannot be dissolved by the human body fluid because the body is saturated with titanium. This is one reason for the inertness of titanium in the body.

In the case of contact problems without relative motion (see also above the comments on wear) the concentration of electrolytes in small gaps can theoretically cause local crevice corrosion. Clinical practice has shown that this is clinically not relevant for titanium.

CLINICAL ASPECTS

Titanium plates and screws

Clinical experience with pure titanium and titanium alloys exists for more than 20 years, and has proven that there are no biological problems. Titanium wear particles may show dark color and may sometimes lead to discussions for cosmetic reasons. Only in the case of unstable osteosyntheses with thin soft tissue cover may there be a visible effect.

In 1975 T.Rüedi [8] performed a study on the clinical use of titanium and investigated the "mixing" of titanium plates with stainless steel screws. No negative clinical effect was observed after various implantation periods. If a fracture fixation is loose there may be fretting corrosion and wear. This is undesirable. In general dissimilar metals should not be combined in plate and screw systems.

Plate contouring of stainless steel plates

A study by Frankle et al.[4] on 500 documented cases on plates has shown that the maximum of strain applied by plate contouring in standard applications at the tibia to a plate does not exceed 1.6% in average which is far below the elongation at fracture for cp titanium (12%). The total strain applied by contouring can be very easy calculated from the average anatomical curvature of the relevant bone surfaces especially at the condyle area of the long bones (Fig.2). The strain e applied by contouring a straight plate (thickness s) to a diameter D by pure bending is

$$e = s/(D+s) \ . \qquad\qquad (1)$$

The diameter D is determined by the anatomy, the plate thickness s is given by the design (Fig.3).

Handling

If the surgeon performing a contouring does not exceed the above mentioned anatomical values and he does not bend the plate frequently the induced plastic strain will not remarkably reduce the strain limit of the material.

The different stress-strain relationship of titanium compared with stainless steel needs the development of different feel for the insertion of bone screws.

Titanium (and especially titanium alloy) is not always as forgiving as stainless steel. The torque difference between start of plastic deformation and the failure is smaller for titanium than for steel. Additional "wobbling" (that means frequent tilting of the screwdriver axis) may decrease the available load carrying capacity of the material located in the neck of the screw. Therefore, sufficient practice of inserting titanium screws is necessary.

Clinical experience

Recently the Association for the Study of Internal Fixation (ASIF) has started an extensive clinical study with the LC-DCP (Limited contact dynamic compression plate). The plates are made from AO/ASIF cp titanium. Matter et al. [16] first reported on this in 1990. More than 500 cases have been documented now. The preliminary results confirmed the concept and were published in 1993 [17]. From this study further conclusions will be drawn for the future application of cp Titanium in internal fixation [18].

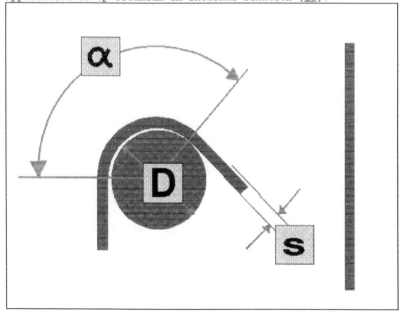

FIG.3-- Strain caused by contouring of plates

CONCLUSION

Unalloyed titanium has proven good biocompatibility and is standardized in ISO 5832-2. The mechanical properties are equivalent to stainless steel, certain differences exist which may need certain changes in design and different handling by the surgeon.

Increasing allergic reactions to metals (nickel, chrom) and the higher risk of complications in the case of allergy indicate a move away from stainless steel. Toxic alloy components should be avoided whenever feasible. They are not critical in the case of stable fixations but they can produce toxic ions if local relative motion between implant components occurs. Pure titanium performs better in such critical cases.

REFERENCES
[1] Lane, W.A.: The operative treatment of fractures, London, The Medical Publishing C., 1914
[2] Lambotte , A.: Les débits de L'osteosynthése en Belgique. Ed. Société Belge de chirurgie orthoped. et de Traumotologie 1921 1971, Bruxelles, 1971
[3] Beder, O.E.; Eade, G.: An investigation of tissue tolerance to titanium metal implants in dogs. Surgery 39, p.470-473, 1956.
[4] Frankle, M.A.; Cordey, J.; Frankle, M.D.; Baumgart, F.; Perren, S.M.: A Retrospective Analysis of Plate Contouring in the Tibia using the conventional 4.5mm (narrow) DC Plate, J. of Orthop.Trauma, submitted 1991, to be published in 1993.
[5] Steinemann, S.G.; Mäusli, P.-A.; Szmukler-Moncler, S.; Semlitsch, M.; Pohler, O.;Hintermann, H.-E.; Perren, S.M.: Beta-Titanium Alloy for Surgical Implants , paper presented at the Seventh World Conference on Titanium, June 1992, San Diego
[6] Perren, S. et al.: Biomaterials conf., Paris, 1987.
[7] ISO 5832-2 Implants for Surgery - Metallic Materials - Part II : Unalloyed Titanium, International Organization for Standardization, Geneva, Switzerland
[8] Rüedi, Th.P.: Titan und Stahl in der Knochenchirurgie, Hefte zur Unfallheilkunde, Heft 123, Springer-Verlag, Berlin Heidelberg New York, 1975
[9] ISO 5832-3 Implants for Surgery - Metallic Materials - Part 3: Wrought titanium 6 aluminum 4 vanadium alloy, International Organization for Standardization, Geneva, Switzerland
[10] ISO DIS 5832-11 Implants for Surgery - Metallic Materials - Part 11 : Titanium 6 aluminum 7 niobium alloy, Draft International Standard 1993, International Organization for Standardization, Geneva, Switzerland
[11] ISO 5832-10 Implants for Surgery - Metallic Materials - Part 10: Titanium 5 aluminum 2.5 ironalloy, International Organization for Standardization, Geneva, Switzerland

[12] Frey, N.; Buchillier,T.; Le, V.-D.; Steinemann, S.G.: Properties of surface oxides on titanium and some titanium alloys, paper presented at the Seventh World Conference on Titanium, June 1992, San Diego

[13] Gerber, H.; Perren, S.: "Evaluation of Tissue Compatibility of in vitro Cultures of Embryonic Bone", in Evaluation of Biomaterials, John Wiley & Sons Ltd., 1980, pp.307-314

[14] Hierholzer,S. and G.: Osteosynthese und Metallallergie - Klinische Untersuchungen, Immunologie und Histologie des Implantatlagers, in: Traumatologie aktuell, Georg Thieme Verlag Stuttgart, New York 1991

[15] Steinemann, S.G.: Personal communication, 1992.

[16] Matter, P. et al. in: AO/ASIF Poster exhibition at SICOT 1990, Montreal, Canada.

[17] Matter et al.: Annual meeting of the Swiss Society of Surgery, Davos, 1993

[18] Allgöwer,M.; Müller,M.E.; Schneider,R; Willenegger,H.: Manual of internal fixation, third edition, Springer, 1991

J. A. Disegi[1] and D. M. Cesarone[2]

METALLURGICAL PROPERTIES OF UNALLOYED TITANIUM
LIMITED CONTACT DYNAMIC COMPRESSION PLATES

REFERENCE: Cesarone, D. M., and Disegi, J. A., "Metallurgical
Properties of Unalloyed Titanium Limited Contact Dynamic
Compression Plates," Clinical and Laboratory Performance of Bone
Plates, ASTM STP 1217, J. P. Harvey, Jr., and R. F. Games, Eds.,
American Society for Testing and Materials, Philadelphia, 1994.

ABSTRACT: The AO/ASIF Limited Contact Dynamic Compression Plate
(LC-DCP®) is fabricated from implant quality unalloyed titanium material
that conforms to ASTM F67 standard [1]. Broad and narrow 4.5 mm plates
and small 3.5 mm plates are used with unalloyed titanium bone screws for
fracture fixation of the femur, tibia, and forearm. The LC-DCP concept
of biological plating is described elsewhere.

Metallurgical properties must be closely controlled to provide a
satisfactory level of functional performance. Microstructure,
composition, processing, and testing guidelines are important for bone
plate applications. Optimum microstructure features include fine grain
size, absence of nonmetallic inclusions, and low volume fraction of TiFe
intermetallic phase. The influence of iron on the corrosion resistance
of unalloyed titanium is well documented.

Special metallurgical processing ensures an enhanced combination
of strength and ductility. Bone plate raw material is evaluated
according to a standardized bend test method. Four point bend testing
data is compared for titanium LC-DCP and 316L stainless steel DCP
implants.

KEYWORDS: unalloyed titanium, bone plate, tensile strength,
microstructure, corrosion, bending strength, bending rigidity

---

Biological bone plating concepts have been incorporated into the
design of the the AO/ASIF Limited Contact Dynamic Compression Plate (LC-
DCP). These plates are primarily used for fracture fixation of the femur
tibia, and forearm. Major elements of the LC-DCP design are described
elsewhere [2]. Unalloyed titanium LC-DCP and 316L stainless steel DCP
implants that have been slightly contoured are shown in Fig. 1. A key
feature of this biological plating system has been the selection of
unalloyed titanium implant material for the bone plates and screws.
The excellent biocompatibility of unalloyed titanium has been well
documented in the literature [3].

---

[1]Materials Development Director and [2]Mechanical Test Engineer,
respectively, SYNTHES (USA), Paoli, PA. 19301.

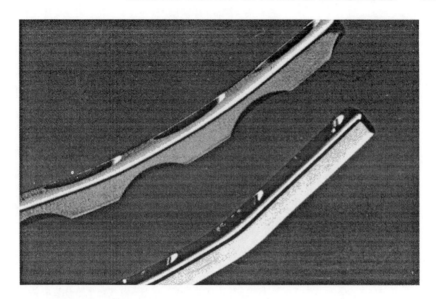

FIG. 1-- Side view of contoured titanium LC-DCP (top) and 316L
stainless DCP (bottom) implants.

Proper control of essential metallurgical properties are necessary to
ensure acceptable functional performance of titanium bone plates.
A satisfactory level of compositional uniformity, microstructure
homogeneity, and predictable mechanical behavior are crucial. The
objective of the present study was to document the major attributes that
have a pronounced effect on the metallurgical quality of unalloyed
titanium LC-DCP material. Static four point bend testing of typical
3.5 mm and 4.5 mm bone plate designs were performed according to ISO
9585 [4].

MICROSTRUCTURE CONTROL

The composition of unalloyed titanium or commercially pure (CP)
implant material is specified in ASTM F 67 industry standard. Double or
triple vacuum melting produces a single phase alpha microstructure that
is free of nonmetallic inclusions. Metallographic examination at 100X
magnification typically reveals a complete absence of inclusions.
However, refractory metal and nitrogen stabilized Type I alpha
inclusions have been identified [5] in CP grades. The refractory metal
or High Density Inclusion (HDI) may contain high melting point
contaminants such as tungsten, tungsten carbide, molybdenum, tantalum,
etc. Weldments, mixed scrap, and machine tool fragments are possible
sources of contamination. Nitrogen stabilized Type I alpha also known as
Low Density Inclusion (LDI) is an intermetallic compound of titanium and
nitrogen. Raw material, electrode fabrication or air contamination
during melting are major sources of Type I alpha. Primary titanium
suppliers rely on raw material control and sophisticated melting
technology to minimize these types of undesirable inclusions.

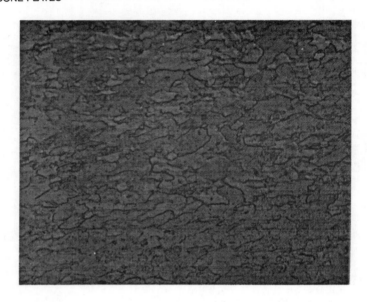

FIG. 2--Transverse microstructure of unalloyed titanium bone plate
stock at 250X magnification.

The transverse microstructure of unalloyed titanium bone plate stock
(Fig. 2) shows a fine grain equiaxed structure with an ASTM 7.5 grain
size rating according to ASTM E112 method [6]. A uniformly fine grain
size rating is important to achieve a good combination of strength
and ductility.

The microstructure of unalloyed titanium can be altered by various
metallurgical treatments. An annealed microstructure is obtained by
heating the material to a defined temperature of around 700°C followed
by a specific cooling cycle. Cold working can also be used to strengthen
the titanium by deforming the material at room temperature while thermal
stress relieving treatments will equalize the stress distribution
throughout the cross section. Superior microstructures can be obtained
for unalloyed titanium depending on the degree of deformation and
thermal handling guidelines that are specified.

A residual amount of iron in the form of TiFe is usually present
[7] as an intermetallic compound. The influence of iron content on
corrosion resistance can be significant. Low iron content has been shown
to improve the stability of the protective oxide film. Unalloyed
titanium with a low iron content of 0.020% has demonstrated a 40%
increase in anodic breakdown potential in 3.5% sodium chloride at 25°C
when compared to a composition containing 0.150% iron [8].

Iron contamination on the surface of titanium or the presence of
iron in the microstructure can also decrease the corrosion resistance in
reducing acids. Accelerated laboratory tests have documented (Fig. 3) a
threefold difference in the corrosion rate of unalloyed titanium as a
function of iron content when exposed to a reducing acid solution [8].
Unalloyed titanium compositions with low iron content should be
specified to ensure that maximum corrosion resistance will be
maintained.

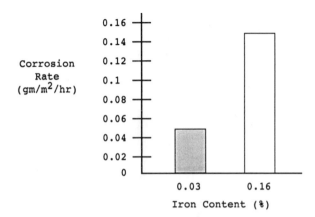

FIG. 3--Effect of iron content on the corrosion rate of
unalloyed titanium in 10% hydrochloric acid (HCl) at 21°C.
(RMI Co., Niles, OH).

Hydrogen content must be kept very low in titanium compositions to
avoid hydrogen embrittlement. Titanium cleaning operations which use
nitric-hydrofluoric acid solutions must be carefully controlled to
eliminate hydrogen absorption during pickling. A ratio of 10 parts
nitric acid to 1 part hydrofluoric acid is recommended [9].

MECHANICAL PROPERTIES

Refined titanium compositions that are processed in a controlled
manner can yield significant improvements in mechanical properties.
The minimum tensile strength and minimum elongation for selected grades
of unalloyed titanium are compared in Fig. 4. The minimum tensile
strength for cold worked Grade 4B titanium bar is 680 MPa with a minimum
10% elongation according to ISO 5832-2 [10] specification. Strength and
ductility minimums can be increased when compared to standard or
industry requirements for moderate strength unalloyed titanium bar
product.

ASTM F 67 specifies minimum 15% elongation plus minimum 550 MPa
tensile strength for Grade 4 and minimum 18% elongation plus minimum 450
MPa for Grade 3 in the annealed condition. Tensile strength can also be
increased without decreasing elongation when high ductility requirements
are needed. Typical mechanical properties will also extend beyond the
minimum tensile strength and ductility values for both standard and
advanced metallurgical conditions.

The mechanical property diagram indicates that specialized
processing results in a significantly greater tensile strength when
compared to conventional processing. Higher strength capabilities and
excellent ductility are achieved as a result of the unique combination
of microstructure control and advanced processing methods. Increased
strength is desirable because of improved resistance to fatigue failure.
High ductility is needed to prevent microcrack development during bone
plate contouring.

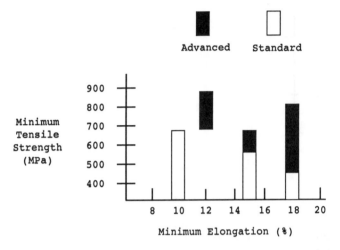

FIG. 4--Minimum tensile properties for unalloyed titanium
       implant material.

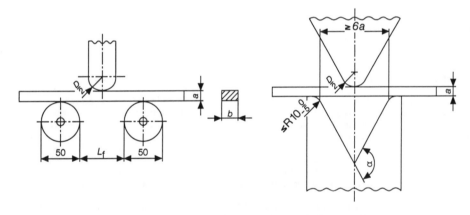

FIG. 5--DIN 50111 bend test arrangement depicting two rollers and
       mandrel (left) or V-block and mandrel (right) prior to testing.

Bend testing of raw material stock used to fabricate LC-DCP
implants is considered an important mechanical property requirement that
must be satisfied. The bending properties are evaluated according to the
methods outlined in DIN 50111 [11]. The bend test arrangement [Fig. 5]
includes a mandrel with either two rollers or a V-block. Regardless of
the method chosen, the major problem is defining appropriate acceptance
and rejection criteria for evaluating cracks after bending the material
to an angle of 105°. ASTM E 190 [12] does not consider cracks occurring
on the corners of the specimen during bend testing unless they exceed a
specified size or show evidence of defects. According to ASTM E 290
[13], the convex surface is inspected for cracks exceeding a specified
number and size unless complete failure occurs.

The actual criteria used to evaluate the bending quality of unalloyed titanium LC-DCP bone plate stock is summarized as follows:

a) Bend test rejection is defined as the occurrence of one or more transverse cracks on the tension side, the length of which is equal to 20% or more of the width dimension, regardless of whether or not the crack originates at the edge. The crack depth is not measured.

b) Surface separation associated with defects such as pinholes, laps, seams, edge defects, etc, are not counted as a bend test failure as long as the defect is localized and does not propagate greater than 20% in the transverse plane after bending.

TABLE 1-- Mean bending strength and stiffness of
AO/ASIF bone plates (n=5).

Design	Material	Mean Bending Strength (Nm)	Mean Bending Stiffness (Nm^2)
3.5 DCP	(316L)	17.3 ± 0.3	3.1 ± 0.1
3.5 LC-DCP	(Ti)	14.5 ± 0.5	1.6 ± 0.1
4.5 Narrow DCP	(316L)	23.3 ± 0.4	5.2 ± 0.3
4.5 Narrow LC-DCP	(Ti)	25.1 ± 1.1	3.9 ± 0.1
4.5 Broad DCP	(316L)	55.1 ± 2.6	12.1 ± 1.5
4.5 Broad LC-DCP	(Ti)	51.1 ± 0.4	9.1 ± 0.1

BONE PLATE BEND TESTING

The four point bending properties of fully finished titanium LC-DCP and 316L stainless DCP implants were evaluated according to the method outlined in ISO 9585. Five plates of each design were tested. Testing was performed with an MTS 810 load frame and model 458 controller. The load versus deflection was recorded on a Yokogawa X-Y chart recorder. The deflection was defined as the change in position of the bottom rollers mounted on the actuator relative to the top rollers mounted on the load cell. The mean bending strength, mean bending stiffness, and standard deviation are compiled (Table 1) for various 3.5 mm and 4.5 mm DCP and LC-DCP bone plates.

The bending strength of the 3.5 mm titanium LC-DCP was approximately 84% of the stainless steel DCP. Titanium LC-DCP stiffness was significantly lower than the stainless DCP. The narrow 4.5 mm LC-DCP bending strength exceeded the bending strength of stainless DCP. LC-DCP stiffness was 74% of the 316L stainless DCP. Broad 4.5 mm plates exhibited similar bending strengths while the stiffness of the titanium LC-DCP was about 72% of the stainless DCP.

Overall results indicated that the titanium LC-DCP design was comparable in bending strength with significantly lower bending stiffness when compared to the stainless DCP. Reduced bending stiffness is expected since the theoretical modulus of elasticity for unalloyed titanium is 55% of implant quality 316L stainless steel. Three different techniques can be used to measure deflection in ISO 9585 depending on the test set-up and bone plate geometry. This will effect the slope of the load versus deflection curve and can influence the equivalent bending stiffness calculations.

Highly localized permanent deformation was observed (Fig.1) for stainless DCP plates when compared to the titanium LC-DCP design. The identical section modulus between the holes and through the holes of the LC-DCP profile provides uniform permanent deformation along the longitudinal axis. By contrast, the stainless steel DCP exhibits localized deformation through the holes because of the reduced section moduli at these locations.

CONCLUSIONS

1. Low density and high density inclusions must be absent in order to eliminate undesirable secondary phases in alpha titanium microstructures.

2. Unalloyed titanium containing a low iron content provides enhanced corrosion resistance in reducing acid and chloride salt solutions.

3. Improved tensile strength and ductility properties may be obtained for unalloyed titanium compositions that are subjected to advanced processing methods.

4. Four point bending results indicate comparable bending strength and lower bending stiffness for titanium LC-DCP bone plates when compared to 316L stainless DCP bone plates.

ACKNOWLEDGEMENT

Dr. L. D. Zardiackas, University of Mississippi Medical Center, Division of Biomaterials, is acknowledged for providing the titanium bone plate micrograph.

REFERENCES

[1]   ASTM F 67 Standard Specification for Unalloyed Titanium for Surgical Implant Applications, American Society for Testing and Materials, Philadelphia, PA.

[2]   Perren, S., Klaue, K., Pohler, O., Predieri, M., Steinemann, S., and Gautier, E., The limited contact dynamic compression plate (LC-DCP), Archives of Orthopaedic and Trauma Surgery, 1990, pp. 304-310.

[3]   Disegi, J., AO/ASIF Unalloyed Titanium Implant Material, Technical Brochure, Second Edition, July 1991, pp. 17-18.

[4]   ISO 9585 Implants for surgery-Method for testing bending strength and stiffness of bone plates, International Organization for Standardization, 1988.

[5]   Shannon, R., Common Types of Segregation or Inclusions in Titanium Alloys, Internal Report, Teledyne Allvac, Monroe, NC.

[6]   ASTM E 112 Test Methods for Determining Average Grain Size, American Society for Testing and Materials, Philadelphia, PA.

[7] Hülse, K., Kramer, K., Breme, J., and Schmidt, D.,
     Influence of small additions of Fe, Cr, and Ni on the
     recrystallization behavior of commercially pure
     titanium, Internal Report, Deutsche Titan Gmbh, Essen,
     West Germany, 1988.

[8] Low iron, commercially pure titanium - a standard
     product of the RMI Company, Technical Brochure, RMI
     Company, Niles, OH.

[9] ASTM B 600 Standard Recommended Practice for Descaling
     and Cleaning Titanium and Titanium Surfaces, American
     Society for Testing and Materials, Philadelphia, PA.

[10] ISO 5832-2 Implants for surgery - Metallic materials -
     Part II: Unalloyed Titanium, International Organization
     for Standardization.

[11] DIN 50111 Bend Test, English Translation, International
     Organization for Standardization, September 1987.

[12] ASTM E 190 Guided Bend Test for Ductility of Welds,
     American Society for Testing and Materials,
     Philadelphia, PA.

[13] ASTM E 290 Semi-Guided Bend Test for Ductility of
     Metallic Materials, American Society for Testing and
     Materials, Philadelphia, PA.

F.W.Baumgart[1], S.M.Perren[2]

THE CONCEPT OF BIOLOGICAL INTERNAL FIXATION USING LIMITED CONTACT PLATES

REFERENCE: Baumgart, F. W., and Perren, S. M., **"The Concept of Biological Internal Fixation Using Limited Contact Plates,"** <u>Clinical and Laboratory Performance of Bone Plates, ASTM STP 1217</u>, J. P. Harvey, Jr., and R. F. Games, Eds., American Society for Testing and Materials, Philadelphia, 1994.

ABSTRACT: The internal fixation of bone fractures aims at early, complete and lasting recovery of limb function. For many years, emphasis was placed on precise reduction and interfragmentary compression as a means of keeping the fragment surfaces from moving. In cases of multifragmentary fractures, this procedure involves extensive surgical intervention and causes additional damage to the circulation of bone. The idea of biological fixation based on the work of Ganz and Mast aims to achieve a sufficiently stable fixation with minimal encroachment on the intact tissue.
 A common phenomenon observed in relation to internal fixation using bone plates is that of temporary porosis beneath the plate. Bone remodelling occurred and infection was liable to cause the formation of a sequestrum.
This porosis was initially explained in mechanical terms as the result of the stress protection function of the plate. Later the work of Gunst, Gautier, Rahn, and Perren et al. demonstrated that the disturbance of blood flow due to compression of the periosteum was the important factor. This has lead to the development of the limited contact dynamic compression plate (LC-DCP). The LC-DCP has proved its worth as an implant which complies with the concept of biological fixation and which has improved the quality of treatment in general.

KEYWORDS: biological internal fixation, limited contact, bone plates, porosis, vascularization, blood flow, necrosis, staining, titanium

[1] Head of AOTK Product Information, Clavadelerstrasse, 7270 Davos Platz, Switzerland
[2] Head of AO Research Institute, Clavadelerstrasse, 7270 Davos Platz, Switzerland

The development of internal fixation

Exact reduction, early loading

Initially internal fixation of fractures was performed with the direct aim of reducing the fragments as exactly as possible. These procedures were based on very sound mechanical principles: An exact fit of the bone fragments provides good bone support and allows one to fix the fracture with relatively small implants and to substitute the missing tensile strength of the bone at the fracture site, while transmission of compression and limited shear stress is still available.

Exact reduction and fixation allow the patient to bear weight early. This supports healing by regular functional use of the limbs and avoids soft tissue atrophy during immobilization. This is one great advantage of stable internal fixation.

The pioneers of internal fixation [1] started systematic application of such techniques using it mainly for simple fractures. The reduction could be performed without dramatic damage to the surrounding soft tissue.

The technique became a "standard" later and naturally the indications expanded to more complicated fractures with much more difficult soft tissue conditions and with far more damage to the bone fragments. The exact reduction and stable fixation of such fractures produced additional destruction to the tissue (vascularization) and to the bone. The fixation was stable, but was detrimental to the bone in some cases, e.g. necrosis.

In both clinical and experimental practice a phenomenon was observed which came to be known as the "stress protection effect" or "stress shielding". This referred to the temporary porosity occurring beneath the plate after a certain implantation period.

The pure mechanistic point of view at that time led to the explanation that the bone needed a certain amount of stress to prevent degeneration. This was in agreement with Wolff's theory of bone remodelling. Detailed investigations later pointed to another explanation [2][3][4][5].

Early temporary porosis

Gunst, Suter and Rahn, [6] investigated the problem in detail and detected the not inconsiderable influence of the local disturbance of blood flow on the porotic degeneration effects under the plate. Perren et al.,[7], summarized and analyzed further work on this subject in a basic paper, describing the concept of limited contact and how this effect could be applied to the development of new plates.

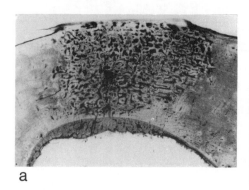
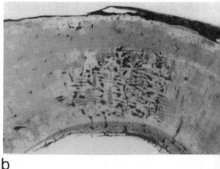

a   b

Fig.1 Temporary porosis under a flat plate
  a) disturbed blood supply under a flat plate
  b) reduced porosis under a plate with small contact
     areas

In comparative in vivo studies on sheep with special
profiled test plates a temporary effect could be reproduced
and observed: Under the flat plate, an area of porous bone
could be detected for a certain time after plating (Fig.1).
     Disulphin blue staining demonstrated the disturbance of
blood flow due to local compression beneath the plate caused
by screw tightening and plate contact. The blood supply to
the peripheral one-third of the cortex is mainly provided k
the periosteum. If the vessels in the periosteum are impede
by pressure, the blood supply will be interrupted and the
bone becomes partially porotic.
     This porosis was found to be temporary and disappeared
again after three to four months. Plates with smaller
contact surfaces did not cause this disturbance of blood
flow or the consequent porosis.
     Stress shielding of the bone may play a role as well,
but has obviously much less influence than the loss of bloc
supply.

The Concept of Limited Contact (LC)

The elements of the LC fixation

The concept of limited contact in the plating of
fractures is based on the results of these investigations.
The advantages of limited contact plating are observed
locally, i.e. in the vicinity of the applied device. The
concept of LC applied to a plate consists of the following
three elements:
        - small contact areas at the undersurface of the plate
        - pure titanium for optimal biological conditions
        - optimized variable profile to provide uniform
stiffness and strength.

The use of pure titanium and the optimization of design are found to be essential to provide higher biological and technical safety.

<u>The properties of the plate</u>

For the development of the AO Limited Contact Dynamic Compression Plate (LC-DCP) the following elements have been additionally introduced
- trapezoidal cross section of the plate for easy removal
- symmetric equidistant holes to allow compression in two directions, investigated by KLAUE [9]
- the possibility of inclination of the screws is increased in both planes.

The plate has undercuts beneath the plate which reduce the contact area between bone and plate to a minimum (limited contact) (Fig.2). The upper surface of the plate has grooves. Extended FEM studies done by GASSER led to the final optimized design with uniform bending and torsional stiffness and uniform strength [8].

Other observed effects, such as the tendency of the newly formed bone to build a bed for the plate and the difficulty of uniformly contouring the plate without large local deformations at the (weak) screw holes also called for design optimization of the 25 year old Dynamic Compression Plate (DCP).

Progress in biomaterials development enables us to recommend cp titanium for internal fixation implants for two reasons:
- pure titanium is free from known side effects. Allergic reactions have not been reported. We can assume that this material is the best available metallic material for internal fixations today.
- Implants for fracture fixation in general have to be removed after 1 to 2 years. However, in some cases it may be desirable to leave the implant in situ because the patient's condition is weak or the patient may not wish to have the implant removed.

Titanium offers the advantage that it can be left in the body indefinitely which is not necessarily true for stainless steel implants.

The concept of biological fixation

<u>What does "biological" fixation mean?</u>

"Biological" fixation is a new general concept in surgical technique for internal fixation. It takes the optimal biomechanical stability and minimal disturbance of the biological environment of the fracture into consideration. In comparison with the concept of LC, biological fixation is a general concept taking into account the whole fracture situation including soft tissue damage. Reduction and number of implants should be kept to a safe minimum.

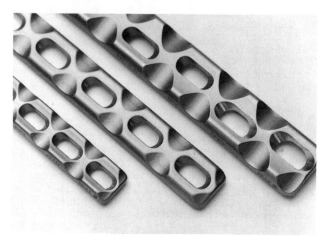

Fig.2   LC-DCP with undercuts

The geometry of the fracture

The geometry of the fracture determines the kind of fixation. If the fracture is very complex, the fixation will also be complicated in most cases. A simple oblique fracture could be fixed with only one straight plate with 6 or 7 holes, for example.

On the other hand, comminuted fractures may require long plates with many holes and frequently additional lag screws or special plates. It is evident that as the number of implants increases so does the additional damage caused by surgery. In severe, comminuted fractures with extensive tissue damage, biological fixation methods may accelerate the healing process.

Simple vs multifragmented fractures

The development of surgical internal fixation techniques over the last 30 years has greatly expanded the application of devices developed for simple fractures to include more complex surgical indications. A comminuted fracture has completely different biomechanical properties to a simple fracture. In a simple fracture each displacement between the two fragments has to be transmitted over a single gap. This means that the local strain in fibers bridging the gap is high. Two or more fracture gaps (assuming the same width for all gaps) expanded by the same total displacement induces less strain in the newly formed tissue.

Following the strain theory further: A wide gap induces less strain in a fiber (bridging the gap) than an exactly reduced gap if any motion occurs caused by insufficiently stable fixation ! For this reason, an imperfect reduction involving larger gaps may have a positive effect on bone healing (if stable fixation is achieved and only small deformations of the fixation device lead to small relative motion in the gaps!).

Indirect reduction and positioning (angles)

Direct reduction in an open procedure may cause more damage to the soft tissue than an indirect reduction using fracture tables and the image intensifier. Indirect reduction is one aspect of biological fixation [10].

Biological fixation foregoes a perfect reduction. However, there is a need for exact alignment of the bone fragment axes. Additional rotational adjustment is also inevitable.

Partial support by implants and early callus

If the reduction is not perfect and the number of implants (screws) is reduced to a minimum, the fixation is not absolutely stable. The support offered by the implant is only partial. Therefore, weight bearing must be limited to a safe level taking into account the process of healing and bone formation. Early callus formation can be regarded as an additional support allowing partial weight bearing at an early stage of healing. The surgeon has to set the limits for functional loading.

Conventional and bio"logical" technique - a contradiction?

Two variables allow us to categorize and to distinguish conventional and biological techniques:
- the stability of the fracture and the fixation respectively, and
- the damage (preoperative and postoperative).

Fig. 3 shows a very simplified view of the situation of a simple fracture which can be treated using a conventional procedure without causing any significant damage and leading to a nearly stable fixation.

A comminuted fracture can also be treated conventionally; a stable fixation is achieved, but additional damage to the tissue may occur. The threshold for necrosis is exceeded and complications caused by necrotic tissue can be expected.

A bio"logical" fixation tries to stay below the limit of necrosis and still reach maximum stability (or a minimum of instability). The result in general may be much better. This technique is demanding and needs experienced surgeons. Nonetheless, this is a new approach and promises interesting new developments.

The role of the LC-DCP in biological fixation

The use of the LC-DCP for biological internal fixation
is a logical consequence of the new approach. The LC-DCP
supports the idea of biological fixation in terms of its
impingement on the blood supply to the tissues adjacent to
the plate.

Biological Strategy of Fracture Fixation
Bio"logic" vs conventional internal fixation

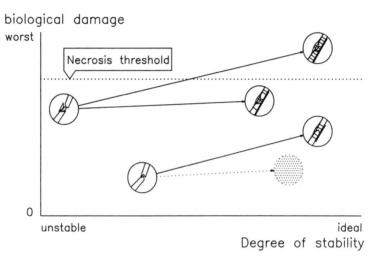

Fig.3   **Comparison of conventional and biological fixation**

Clinical application

Since 1989, the AO/ASIF has been carrying out a
multicentric clinical study on the LC-DCP. The AO
Documentation Center in Davos has documented more than 500
cases to date. The results will be presented this year at
the annual meeting of the Swiss Society of Surgery in Davos.
In 1990, the first results were reported by Matter et al.
[11] (approx. 200 cases). They all showed undisturbed bone
healing and no infections.

The LC-DCP has been designed to meet the requirements
of biological fixation. Its optimized mechanical properties
allow uniform contouring. The surgical technique for
application has not been changed in comparison to the DCP
technique. Only the drill guides had to be modified to fit
the new dimensions of the plate holes.

CONCLUSION

Biological fixation is more demanding for the surgeon than conventional techniques. A clear understanding of the biomechanical situation of the fracture helps to find the right solution for fixation. There is no contradiction between conventional and biological fixation, but this new concept offers the possibility of extending the borders of internal fixation. The LC-DCP as the embodiment of the concept of limited contact is a modern tool offering new opportunities in the treatment of complex fractures and is intended to reduce the complication rate associated with conventional treatment procedures.

REFERENCES

[1] Allgöwer,M., Müller,M.E., Schneider,R., Willenegger,H., Manual der Osteosynthese, 1.Auflage, Springer-Verlag, 1960.
[2] Gautier,E., Cordey,J., Mathys,R., Rahn,B.A., Perren,S.M., Porosity and remodeling of plated bone after internal fixation: result of stress shielding or vascular damage, Elsevier, Amsterdam, 1984.
[3] Jörger,K.A., Akute intrakortikale Durchblutungsstörung unter Osteosyntheseplatten mit unterschiedlichen Auflageflächen. Inaugural dissertation, Bern, 1987.
[4] Perren,S.M., Ganz,R., Rüter,A. Oberflächliche Knochenresorption um Implantate. Medizinische-Orthopadische Technik, 95 (1975), p.6-10.
[5] Gautier,E.R., Rahn,B.A.,Perren,S.M., Effect of steel versus composite plastic plates on internal and external remodeling of intact long bones. Orthop.Trans 10 1986, 391.
[6] Gunst,M.A., Suter,C., Rahn,B.A. "Die Knochendurchblutung nach Plattenosteosynthese. Eine Untersuchung an der intakten Kaninchentibia mit Disulfinblau-Vitalfaerbung", Helvetica Chirurgica Acta 46:171,1979.
[7] Perren,S.M., Cordey,J., Rahn,B.A., Gautier,,E., Schneider,E.: Early Temporary Porosis of Bone Induced by Internal Fixation Implants, Clinical Orthopaedics and Related Research, 232 (7/1988),139 ff.
[8] Gasser,B., Doctoral thesis, University of Basel, 1989.
[9] Klaue,K., The dynamic compression unit (DCU) for stable internal fixation of bone fractures. Doctoral thesis, Basel, 1989.
[10] Mast,J., Jakob,R., Ganz,R., Planning and reduction technique in fracture surgery, Springer, Berlin Heidelberg New York, 1989.
[11] AO/ASIF Poster exhibition, SICOT 1990, Montreal.

Testing Methods

Ajit Nazre[1] and Steve Lin[1]

THEORETICAL STRENGTH COMPARISON OF BIOABSORBABLE (PLLA) PLATES AND CONVENTIONAL STAINLESS STEEL AND TITANIUM PLATES USED IN INTERNAL FRACTURE FIXATION

REFERENCE: Nazre, A., and Lin, S., "Theoretical Strength Comparison of Bioabsorbable (PLLA) Plates and Conventional Stainless Steel and Titanium Plates Used in Internal Fracture Fixation," Clinical and Laboratory Performance of Bone Plates, ASTM STP 1217, J. P. Harvey, Jr., and R. F. Games, Eds., Amercian Society for Testing and Materials, Philadelphia, 1994.

ABSTRACT: Use of stainless steel or titanium plates with multiple screws to fix fractures internally is the most widely used technique in orthopaedics. Metal plates act as a bridge across the fracture gap and stress shield the fracture site as the bone heals. However, use of metal plates in certain applications can be slightly disadvantageous. Due to the high stiffnesses of metal plates they tend to stress shield the fracture site, which can lead to over all reduction of strength of the healing bone. Also, a secondary surgery has to be performed to retrieve the implant, which can increase the risk to the patient. Use of bioabsorbable plates can overcome these disadvantages. This study compares theoretical bending (four point) strengths of three bioabsorbable poly L-lactic acid (PLLA) plates with a stainless steel plate with four holes and four screws. Three types of bioabsorbable plates have been considered, namely, 1. pure PLLA plate, 2. PLLA with glass fibers, and 3. PLLA with carbon fibers. A strength degradation curve for PLLA has been established.

KEYWORDS: Bone plates, Bioabsorbable, Bending Strength, Degradation properties

---

INTRODUCTION: There are three methods of fracture fixation available to the orthopaedic surgeon, namely, 1. closed, 2. open with a variety of implants, and 3. a combination of 1 and 2. The first reported use of the open technique with plates as implants was in 1886 by Hannsman. Most of the plates used now are of the self-compression type, i.e. they compress the fracture fragments into bony apposition as the screws are driven into the bone. When a plate is applied without interfragmentary compression, physical activity produces motion between fracture fragments, thus stimulating resorption of bone at the opposing ends of the fragments. This leads to instability. Loss of bony contact and support can cause fatigue failure of the plates in use.

---

[1]Development Engineer and Director, Advanced Technology respectively, ⁊er, Inc., P.O. Box 708, Warsaw, IN 46581-0708.

The three main functions of a bone plate in internal fixation are: buttressing, neutralization, and compression. Since plates have to withstand high bending moments, plates should be designed with optimum bending strength and stiffness. A very stiff plate could result in stress shielding of the bone underneath the plate and could lead to disuse osteoporosis. This is a major concern in using metal plates. Possible corrosion of metal and surgery for implant retrieval could be enumerated as some other disadvantages of using metal plates.

In order to address these concerns associated with metallic bone plates, other materials such as partially or fully bioabsorbable composites have been considered in the recent past [5]. A bioabsorbable polymer such as poly L-lactic acid (PLLA) could be used as a matrix material along with carbon or glass fibers to form excellent composites. PLLA is an excellent bioabsorbable thermoplastic polymer and it undergoes hydrolytic deesterification to form metabolites normally found in the body. Another major advantage of PLLA is that its degradation can be controlled. Carbon fibers are extremely biocompatible and inert, but are not bioabsorbable. Glass fibers can be bioabsorbable if they are formulated from calcium phosphates [1,2]. E-glass fibers are used in this study because of the availability of the physical mechanical properties.

The main objectives of this study are:

i. To calculate the theoretical bending strength of three types of bioabsorbable plates, namely, 1. pure PLLA plate, 2. PLLA / Glass fiber plate, and 3. PLLA / Carbon fiber plate;

ii. To establish strength degradation curves for the bioabsorbable plates;

iii. To compare bending strengths of the three types of bioabsorbable plates with those of stainless steel and Titanium plates.

METHODS AND MATERIALS

Biomechanics of Plating: As mentioned previously, the three main purposes of a bone plate are buttressing, neutralization and compression. Plating provides static compression of fragments and interfragmentary friction to oppose shearing forces which would otherwise induce large bending moments and torques on the plate. Restoration of anatomic continuity of fracture fragments is another important aspect of bone plating. Bending and torsion are the most significant loading modalities in the case of a bone plate application. Lawrence et.al. [3] have studied the loads sustained by a bone plate on a human tibia. They determined the strength and rigidity of commercially available plates in bending. They defined 5% permanent angular deformation as failure.

Mechanical Behavior of Composite Laminates: Two approaches can be taken to model the mechanical behavior of composites, namely, micromechanics approach and macromechanics approach [6]. Micromechanics is the study of composite material behavior wherein the interaction of the constituent materials is examined on a local basis. Macromechanics, on the other hand, is the study of composite material behavior where the material is presumed homogeneous and the effects of the constituent materials are detected only as averaged apparent properties of the composite. In the present study, a macromechanics approach has been adopted to model the bending strength of the composite laminate (bone plate).

<u>Micromechanics of a Lamina</u>: The mechanical properties of a lamina are determined by fiber orientation. Figure 1 shows a typical laminate coordinate system, where the length of the beam is in the x-direction and the width of the beam in y-direction. The principal fiber direction is 1 and 2 is normal to that. A counterclockwise rotation of the 1-2 system yields a positive ϕ and a clockwise rotation yields a negative ϕ.

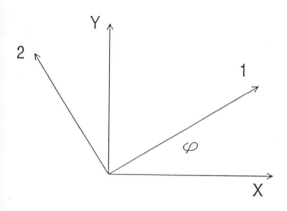

Figure 1 Laminate Coordinate System

The mechanical properties of the lamina are also dependent on the material properties and the volume content of the constituent materials. The equations for the mechanical properties of a lamina in the 1-2 directions are presented below [4].

$$E_1 = E_f V_f + E_m V_m \tag{1}$$

$$E_2 = \frac{E_f E_m}{V_m E_f + V_f E_m} \tag{2}$$

$$v_{12} = V_m v_m + V_f v_f \tag{3}$$

$$v_{21} E_1 = v_{12} E_2 \tag{4}$$

$$G_{12} = \frac{G_f G_m}{V_m G_f + V_f G_m} \tag{5}$$

$$\alpha_{11} = \frac{\alpha_f E_f V_f + \alpha_m E_m V_m}{E_f V_f + E_m V_m} \tag{7}$$

$$\alpha_{22} = \alpha_f V_f (1-\nu_f) + \alpha_m V_m (1-\nu_m) - \alpha_{11}(\nu_f V_f - \nu_m V_m) \tag{6}$$

$$V_m = (1-V_f) \tag{8}$$

where,
E_f = Young's modulus of the fiber
E_m = Young's modulus of the matrix
G_f = Shear modulus of the fiber
G_m = Shear modulus of the matrix
V_f = Volume fraction of the fiber
V_m = Volume fraction of the matrix
ν_f = Poisson's ratio of the fiber
ν_m = Poisson's ratio of the matrix
α_f = Coefficient of thermal expansion of the fiber
α_f = Coefficient of thermal expansion of the matrix.

Macromechanics of a Lamina:
The generalized Hooke's law can be stated as follows:

$$\sigma_i = C_{ij} \epsilon_j \qquad i,j = 1,2,..,6 \tag{9}$$

where,
σ_i = stress components
C_{ij} = Stiffness matrix
ϵ_j = strain components.
(9) can also be expressed as:

$$\epsilon_i = S_{ij} \sigma_j \qquad i,j = 1,2,..,6 \tag{10}$$

where S_{ij} = compliance matrix.
The assumptions made in this analysis are as follows:
i.   The lamina is macroscopically homogeneous, linearly elastic, orthotropic and initially stress free,
ii. The fibers are homogeneous, linearly elastic, isotropic regularly spaced and perfectly aligned, and
iii. The matrix is homogeneous, linearly elastic and isotropic.
Assuming a plane stress condition (9) and (10) reduce to the following:
where Q_{ij} are the reduced stiffnesses, τ_{12} is the shear stress, and ψ_{12} is the shear strain. The equations for the transformation of stresses in the 1-2 direction to the x-y direction are:
where $[T^{-1}]$ is given as;
where, $c=\cos\phi$ and $s=\sin\phi$.

$$
\begin{bmatrix} \epsilon_1 \\ \epsilon_2 \\ \gamma_{12} \end{bmatrix} = \begin{bmatrix} S_{11} & S_{12} & 0 \\ S_{21} & S_{22} & 0 \\ 0 & 0 & S_{66} \end{bmatrix} \begin{bmatrix} \sigma_1 \\ \sigma_2 \\ \tau_{12} \end{bmatrix}
\tag{11}
$$

$$
\begin{bmatrix} \sigma_1 \\ \sigma_2 \\ \tau_{12} \end{bmatrix} = \begin{bmatrix} Q_{11} & Q_{12} & 0 \\ Q_{21} & Q_{22} & 0 \\ 0 & 0 & Q_{66} \end{bmatrix} \begin{bmatrix} \epsilon_1 \\ \epsilon_2 \\ \gamma_{12} \end{bmatrix}
\tag{12}
$$

$$
\begin{bmatrix} \sigma_x \\ \sigma_y \\ \tau_{xy} \end{bmatrix} = [\, T^{-1}\,] \begin{bmatrix} \sigma_1 \\ \sigma_2 \\ \tau_{12} \end{bmatrix}
\tag{13}
$$

$$
[\, T^{-1}] = \begin{bmatrix} c^2 & s^2 & -2cs \\ s^2 & c^2 & 2cs \\ cs & cs & c^2 - s^2 \end{bmatrix}
\tag{14}
$$

Three stiffness matrices [4] are further defined as;

$$
[A_{ij}] = \sum_{k=1}^{N} Q_{ij}{}^k (h_k - h_{k-1})
\tag{15}
$$

$$
[B_{ij}] = \frac{1}{2} \sum_{k=1}^{N} Q_{ij}{}^k (h_k{}^2 - h^2{}_{k-1})
\tag{16}
$$

$$
[D_{ij}] = \frac{1}{3} \sum_{k=1}^{N} Q_{ij}{}^k (h_k{}^3 - h^3{}_{k-1})
\tag{17}
$$

where, $[A_{ij}]$ represents extensional stiffnesses, $[B_{ij}]$ coupling stiffnesses, and $[D_{ij}]$ bending stiffnesses respectively. "k" is the number of lamina in the laminate with maximum N laminae. "h" represents the distance from the neutral axis to the edge of the respective lamina. A standard procedure is followed in numbering the laminae, 0 being at the bottom of a plate and the kth lamina at the top [4]. The A,B,D matrices help define the in-plane and bending properties of the laminate;

$$
Q_{ij} = \frac{A_{ij}}{h}
\tag{18}
$$

in plane and
in bending.
For a balanced symmetric homogeneous composite, the effective laminate

$$Q_I = \frac{12D_{ij}}{h^3} \tag{19}$$

properties in plane and in bending can be described as follows:

$$E_x = \frac{Q_{11}Q_{22} - Q^2_{12}}{hQ_{22}} \tag{20}$$

$$E_y = \frac{Q_{11}Q_{22} - Q^2_{12}}{hQ_{11}} \tag{21}$$

$$\nu_{xy} = \frac{Q_{11}}{Q_{22}} \tag{22}$$

$$\nu_{yx} = \frac{Q_{12}}{Q_{11}} \tag{23}$$

$$G_{xy} = \frac{Q_{66}}{h} \tag{24}$$

The University of Delaware has developed a computer program "Comp-Cal" based on the theory discussed above. Comp-Cal has been used in computing the mechanical properties of the various composites in this study.

Theoretical Four-Point Bend Strengths of Plates: The static four point bend strength was calculated for a total deflection y=0.10 mm (ASTM standard F382-86). Figure 2 shows the plate and the loading arrangement. The force F required to deflect the plate to 0.10mm was calculated using the equation;

$$EI = \frac{(3a^2L - 4a^3)\ F}{6y} \tag{25}$$

where a=40mm and L=120mm and I is the area moment of inertia of the plate defined as;

$$I = \frac{wt^3}{12} \tag{26}$$

where t=thickness of plate (mm), and w=width of plate (mm).

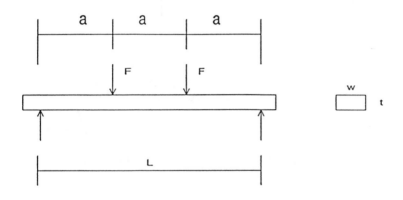

Figure 2 Four Point Bend Test Loading Regime

The theoretical bending strength (bending moment) as defined in ASTM standard F382-86 was then calculated as follows:

$$M = F\,a \tag{27}$$

Theoretical Bending Stiffness of Plates: ASTM standard F382-86 defines bending stiffness (K) of a plate as following,

$$K = \frac{5}{324}\ a^3 \left(\frac{F}{y}\right) \tag{28}$$

Bone Plate Design: A typical AO (Arbeitsgemeinschaft fur Osteosynthesefragen) six hole broad plate (Figure 3), 103mm long, 16mm wide, 6mm thick, and having a 13mm radius of curvature was chosen for analysis. The composite plate design [7] consisted of the following features:

i. a symmetric balanced design

ii. three ratios of 0° and 45° fiber for the three stacking sequences

iii. $V_f = 0.60$

iv. three stacking sequences were used, one of them being; $[0_3/+45/0/-45/0/+45/0/-45/0/+45/0/-45/0/+45/0/-45/0]_s$.

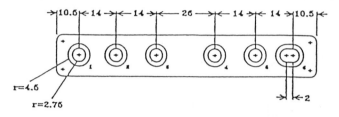

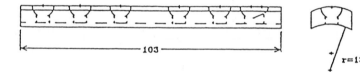

Figure 3 AO Six Hole Broad Plate   * all dimensions in mm.

Material Properties:

Table 1 Material Properties of Constituents [5]

	E_1 (GPa)	E_2 (GPa)	G_{12} (GPa)	G_{22} (GPa)	ν_{12}
316-L SST	193.0	193.0	76.0	76.0	0.27
Ti6A14V	110.0	110.0	42.7	42.7	0.31
PLLA	3.7	3.7	4.0	4.0	0.35
Carbon fiber	207.0	21.0	27.6	6.9	0.20
E-Glass fiber	68.9	68.9	30.0	30.0	0.22

RESULTS AND DISCUSSION

Three types of plates were considered as previously mentioned, namely, pure PLLA, PLLA/E-glass, and PLLA/Carbon (T700). Three different stacking sequences were used in the analysis;

I. $[0_3/+45/0/-45/0/+45/0/-45/0/+45/0/-45/0/+45/0/-45/0]_s$. (38 layers) 60/40 ratio of 0° and 45° fibers.

II. $[0_6/+45/0/-45/0/+45/0/-45/0]_s$. (28 layers) 70/30 ratio of 0° and 45° fibers.

III. $[0_6/+45/0/-45/0]_s$. (20 layers) 80/20 ratio of 0° and 45° fibers.

Three ratios of 0° and 45° fibers were selected. 0° fibers offer higher bending and axial stiffness and 45° fibers contribute to increase in shear modulus. An optimum ratio would offer both bending and shear stiffness. Table 2 presents the mechanical properties of the three plates along with those of the Titanium and Stainless steel plates. Bending strengths computed can also be seen in Table 2.

Table 2. Theoretically Predicted Mechanical Properties of Plates

Material	E_1 (GPa)	E_2 (GPa)	G_{12} (GPa)	ν_{12}	K (Nmm^2)	M (Nm)
Ti6A14V	110	110	42.7	0.31	585	2.37
316-L SST	193	193	76	0.27	1029	4.17
Pure PLLA	37	37	4	0.35	20	0.08
PLLA/E-GF (I)	37.1	19.4	11.8	0.23	198	0.80
PLLA/E-GF (II)	39.6	17.7	11.5	0.24	212	0.86
PLLA/E-GF(III)	41.2	16.7	11.3	0.24	220	0.89
PLLA/CF (I)	94.8	24.6	20.9	0.54	506	2.05
PLLA/CF (II)	109	20.4	17.3	0.50	580	2.35
PLLA/CF (III)	119	17.5	15	0.48	635	2.57

PLLA/E-GF (I) stands for PLLA/E-glass fiber with stacking sequence I and so on. PLLA/CF (I) stands for PLLA/Carbon fiber with stacking sequence (I), etc.

A comparison of the various properties calculated earlier for the different plate materials with respect to the properties of the 316-L stainless steel plate can be seen in Table 3.

Table 3 Comparison of Properties of Plates

Material	E_1 (%)	E_2 (%)	G_{12} (%)	M (%)
Ti6Al4V	56.9	56.9	56.2	56.8
316-L Stainless	100.0	100.0	100.0	100.0
Pure PLLA	19.1	19.1	5.3	1.9
PLLA/E-GF (I)	19.2	10.1	15.5	19.2
PLLA/E-GF (II)	20.5	9.2	15.1	20.6
PLLA/E-GF (III)	21.3	8.6	14.7	21.3
PLLA/CF (I)	49.1	12.7	27.5	49.2
PLLA/CF (II)	56.5	10.6	22.8	56.3
PLLA/CF (III)	61.6	9.1	19.7	61.6

It can be observed that pure PLLA plates with no reinforcement are extremely weak in bending compared to SST (stainless steel) plates. Using E-glass fiber as reinforcement, the bending strength of the PLLA plate increases by about 10.75 times and using carbon fiber the strength is almost 29.3 times higher. In fact, the PLLA/Carbon fiber composite plates are comparable to titanium plates in bending strength. Pure PLLA, PLLA/E-glass fiber and PLLA/Carbon fiber are all significantly more flexible in shear than both SST and titanium.

In case of the reinforced PLLA plates, an increase in bending strength is seen on increasing the ratio of $0°$ and $45°$ fibers. One can account this increase to the longitudinal fibers ($0°$) on the outside of the plate which share the bending stresses. However, increasing this ratio results in a lower shear modulus and hence a lower shear strength.

Based on these observations the partially absorbable PLLA/Carbon fiber plate with stacking sequence (II) appears to be the ideal choice among the various alternatives considered in this study.

<u>Strength Degradation of PLLA</u>: The PLLA polymer considered for application in this study undergoes degradation in tensile strength [5] as seen in Figure 4. There is currently no data available on bending strength degradation of pure PLLA.

Tensile Strength (MPa)

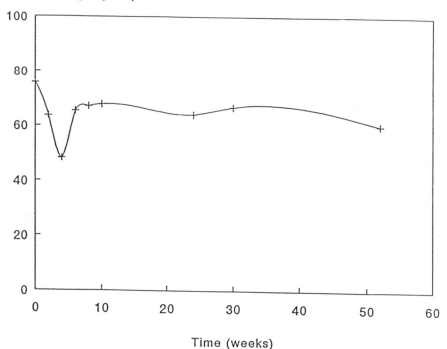

Time (weeks)

Figure 4 Strength Degradation of PLLA

Limitations: Theoretical modeling of the mechanical behavior of composites is a useful tool, but also has certain limitations due to the assumptions made in the analysis. The values of bending strength obtained for the various plate configurations are extremely conservative estimates. Values of bending strength measured experimentally tend to be higher than the ones calculated theoretically, since the theoretical analysis is based on the elastic portion of the moment-displacement curve, as opposed to the elastic-plastic portion for an experimental study. On the other hand, stress concentration due to holes, the manufacturing process used to make these holes can increase or decrease the strength too. These effects are totally overlooked in a theoretical model. The fabrication process of the plates itself lends to a great degree of uncertainty in determining properties. However, ideal conditions are assumed in the theoretical analysis. Torsional loads on the plate have been assumed to be zero for ease of calculation (Plane stress condition), which may not be the case in a real life application. Mechanical behavior in fatigue is also an issue which is better addressed experimentally than theoretically in case of these absorbable composite plates.

Conclusions: Based on the available observations one can conclude that partially and fully absorbable reinforced composite plates are a good alternative to metal plates in areas of low strength applications. Use of bioabsorbable plates in high strength fractures in long weight bearing bones is not recommended from a point of view of strength. On the same token, fully or partially bioabsorbable plates do offer other advantages, such as:
i. minimization of risk by elimination of surgery for retrieval and
ii. reduced stress shielding.

REFERENCES
[1]   Lin, S., "Totally Absorbable Fiber Reinforced Composite for Internal Fracture Fixation Devices", 12th Annual Meeting of the Society of Biomaterials, Minneapolis, MN, May 1986.

[2]   Kumar, B. and Lin, S., "Redox State of Iron and its Related Effects in the $CaO-P_2O_5-Fe_2O_3$ Glasses", Journal of American Ceramic Society, vol. 74, no. 1, pp226-228, 1991.

[3]   Lawrence, M., Freeman, M.A.R., Swanson, S.A., "Engineering Considerations in the Internal Fixation of Fractures of the Tibial Shaft", J.Bone Jt. Surg., 51-B:654, 1969.

[4]   Whitney, J.M., Daniel, I.M., Pipes, R.B., "Experimental Mechanics of Fiber Reinforced Composite Materials", The Society of Experimental Stress Analysis, Brookfield Center, CT., 1982.

[5]   Lin, S., "Poly(L-Lactide Acid) Orthopaedic Fixation Devices", 17th Annual Meeting of the Society of Biomaterials, Scottsdale, AZ, May 1991.

[6]   Tsai, S.W., "Composites Design", Think Composites, Dayton, 1987.

[7]   Zimmermann, M.C., "Design and Analysis of Absorbable and Semi-absorbable Composite Fracture Fixation Devices", Ph.D. Thesis, Rutgers, The State University of New Jersey, 1985.

D. M. Cesarone[1] and J. A. Disegi[2]

TECHNIQUES IN THE APPLICATION OF ISO 9585 TEST METHOD FOR THE DETERMINATION OF BONE PLATE BENDING PROPERTIES

REFERENCE: Cesarone, D. M., and Disegi, J. A., "Techniques in the Application of ISO 9585 Test Method for the Determination of Bone Plate Bending Properties," Clinical and Laboratory Performance of Bone Plates, ASTM STP 1217, J. P. Harvey, Jr. and R. F. Games, Eds., American Society for Testing and Materials, Philadelphia, 1994.

ABSTRACT: Specialized metallic bone plates are used to stabilize various types of bone fractures which occur in the upper and lower extremities. A knowledge of the relative bending strength and stiffness of bone plates is desirable to evaluate the effect of different materials and designs on clinical performance. Bending stiffness in the elastic region is primarily a function of the modulus of elasticity of·the material and plate dimensions. Adequate bending strength is important to resist permanent deformation associated with single-cycle overload stress. Proper contouring of bone plates in the operating room is related to plate design.

ISO 9585, "Implants for Surgery — Method for Testing Bending Strength and Stiffness of Bone Plates," describes a static four-point bend test for bone plates. Testing factors such as bone plate length, cylindrical roller dimensions, and flatness deviations are specified in the ISO test method. Plate placement on the bending rollers and plate orientation must also be controlled for consistent bend test results.

Correct interpretation of the load-deflection curve is required to accurately determine proof load, mean deflection, equivalent bending stiffness, and bending strength. Calculations based on established formulas are presented for typical test configurations.

Bend test results are compiled for implant-quality 316L stainless steel and unalloyed titanium, cloverleaf and T-plates. A modified test arrangement is described for the evaluation of 1.5 mm and 2.0 mm titanium mini-fragment plates.

KEYWORDS: proof load, bending strength, equivalent bending stiffness

The bending properties of small specialized bone plates are important to further our understanding of the strength and stiffness required for fracture stabilization. Specialized metallic bone plates are used primarily to stabilize various types of bone fractures in the upper and lower extremities.

[1]Mechanical Test Engineer and [2]Materials Development Director, respectively, SYNTHES (USA), Paoli, PA. 19301.

A knowledge of the relative bending strength and stiffness of bone plates is desirable to evaluate the effect of different materials and designs on clinical performance. Adequate bending strength is important to resist permanent deformation associated with single-cycle overload stress. Proper contouring of bone plates in the operating room is related to plate design.

The purpose of this study was to evaluate the ISO 9585 test method for determining the static bending strength and equivalent bending stiffness of commonly used AO/ASIF specialized bone plates. The influence of plate geometry and test set-up was also analyzed.

MATERIALS AND METHODS

The implant-quality 316L stainless steel cloverleaf and T-plates were tested in the fully finished, electropolished condition. The unalloyed titanium cloverleaf and T-plates were in the as-machined and tumbled condition, while the titanium mini-fragment plates were anodized. The implant-quality 316L material met the prevailing requirements in ASTM F 139 Grade 2 standard and the unalloyed titanium material conformed to ASTM F 67 specification.

The cloverleaf and T-plates were tested in four-point bending according to ISO 9585 [1] test method. Cylindrical top rollers that measured 12.5 mm diameter were fabricated with contoured central region of variable diameters that match the transverse cross section of the bone plate being tested. Straight 12.5 mm diameter cylindrical rollers were used as bottom supports and mounted to the hydraulic actuator. The top and bottom rollers were restrained in holders to prevent them from moving. The mini-fragment plates were tested according to ISO 9585, except the small dimensions of the plates required the use of 4.0 mm diameter rollers. Each plate was tested one time. All tests were repeated five times (n=5).

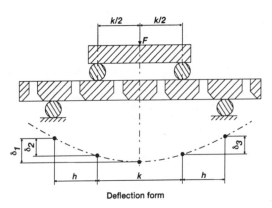

Deflection form

FIG. 1--General arrangement of four-point bend test.

Testing was performed on an MTS 810 load frame with a Model 458 Controller. Loading rate on each bone plate was 1 mm per minute with the bone contact surface facing upward. The load versus deflection was continuously recorded on a Yokogawa X-Y chart recorder. The bending load was applied until sufficient plastic deformation occurred to allow the calculation of the bending strength and stiffness.

The deflection was measured according to section 4.2(i)(1) of ISO 9585. Deflection is defined as the linear displacement due to bending measured perpendicular to the original axis of the plate. The actual deflection may be measured according to three different methods depending on the plate hole geometry. The equivalent bending stiffness was calculated according to the following equation:

$$E = \frac{(4h^2 + 12\ hk + k^2)Sh}{24}$$

Where:

   E is equivalent bending stiffness (Nm^2);
   h is distance between inner and outer rollers (m);
   k is distance between inner rollers (m);
   S is slope of the load versus deflection curve (Nm)

The equivalent bending stiffness equation accounts for the holes in the plate. The load deflection diagram is shown in Figure 2.

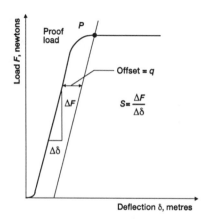

FIG. 2--Load deflection diagram.

The intersection of the load versus deflection curve with the linear offset (q) is defined as the proof load (P). Bending strength is defined as the bending moment at fracture, or a specified proof point, whichever is lower, and is calculated as follows:

$$\text{Bending Strength} = .5\ Ph$$

Where:

   Bending strength is (Nm);
   P is proof load (N);
   h is distance between inner and outer rollers (m)

RESULTS

Proof load, bending strength, and equivalent bending stiffness of the specialized bone plates are shown in Table 1.

Table 1--ISO 9585 Four-Point
Bend Test Results (n=5)

Specimen (MATL)	Proof Load (kN)	Bend Strength (Nm)	Bend Stiffness (Nm^2)
T-Plate (316L)	1.04 ± 0.01	8.33 ± 0.08	1.29 ± 0.22
T-Plate (Ti)	1.19 ± 0.06	9.53 ± 0.05	1.40 ± 0.02
Cloverleaf (316L)	0.39 ± 0.01	3.15 ± 0.05	0.33 ± 0.01
Cloverleaf (Ti)	0.59 ± 0.01	4.72 ± 0.11	0.54 ± 0.01
1.5 mm Mini-Frag. (Ti)	0.09 ± 0.002	0.24 ± 0.006	1.55E-05 ± 4.28E-07
2.0 mm Mini-Frag. (Ti)	0.21 ± 0.002	0.53 ± 0.005	3.56E-05 ± 1.36E-06

The titanium T-plate had a mean proof load about 15% higher than the stainless steel T-plate. The proof load of the titanium cloverleaf plate was about 50% greater than the stainless cloverleaf plate, Figure 3.

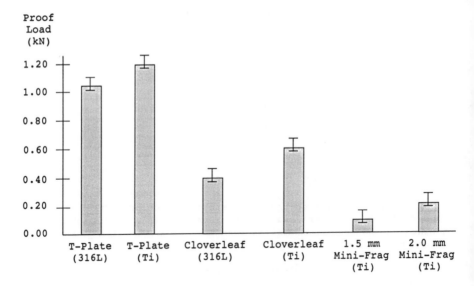

FIG 3--Mean Proof Load of Bone Plates (n=5).

Higher bending stiffness was measured for unalloyed titanium when compared to 316L stainless steel cloverleaf and T-plates. The increased dimensions of the titanium plates more than compensated for the lower modulus of elasticity, Figure 4.

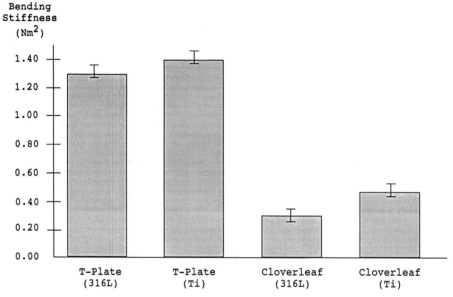

FIG 4-- Bone Plate Mean Equivalent Bending Stiffness (n=5).

Bending strength values for the titanium plates were greater than for the stainless plates, Figure 5.

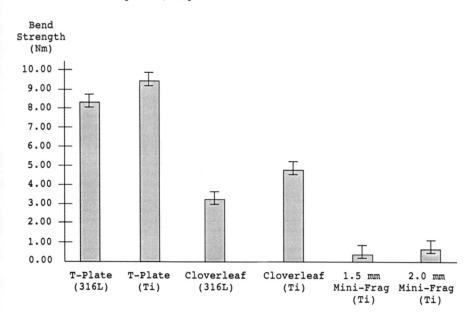

FIG 5-- Bone Plate Mean Bending Strength (n=5).

The titanium mini-fragment plates showed the expected increase in proof load, bending strength, and equivalent bending stiffness for the larger 2.0 mm plate size.

DISCUSSION

Testing factors such as bone plate length, cylindrical roller dimensions, flatness deviations, and plate placement on the bending rollers must be controlled for consistent bend test results. This test procedure is not recommended for plates less than 50 mm in length. The available span length between inner and outer rollers is critical to the mode of loading applied to the plate. An insufficient span length between rollers induces shear stresses on the plate instead of the desired bending load. The test procedure accounts for plate holes. This distributes the applied load over a uniform plate-hole-wall section. The cloverleaf and T-plates could not be tested with the inner rollers placed symmetrically across a uniform cross section. The straight section of the plate was not long enough to allow placement of the plate holes symmetrically on either side of the vertical load axis. Test results are indicative of this.

ISO 9585 specifies a flatness ratio at the center of the plate not to exceed b/6 where b is the width of the plate. Because of plate design and geometry, the cloverleaf and T-plates were tested using rollers whose geometry matched that of the plates' bottom radius. Rollers matching the underside of the bone plate distribute the load over the entire transverse cross section of plate, tangent to that section of roller. Testing plates with a transverse flatness ratio greater than b/6 using straight cylindrical rollers would allow an undistributed load applied to the corners of the plate. The center of the plate would remain unsupported as the load increased. Minute deflection would take place in the longitudinal and transverse planes, thus distorting the recorded load-deflection curve. The geometry of the mini-fragment plates warranted the use of flat cylindrical rollers.

Exact placement of each test specimen onto the test arrangement is critical to the repeatability of the test results. Measuring devices and gauges can be used to position each test specimen in the exact location as the part before it. This ensures that each test part is supported on locations critical to each plate design. This especially holds true when screw hole location is under investigation. Plates positioned in the test stand with the rollers aligned off center to the plate holes will generate an unevenly distributed load along the length of the plate.

Analysis of the bend test results indicated the equivalent bending stiffness of the specialty titanium plates exceeded the stainless plates. The modulus of elasticity (in tension) for unalloyed titanium is about 104 GPa while the modulus for implant-quality 316L stainless is 186 GPa. The lower modulus for titanium was offset by the increased plate dimensions. Bending strength and proof load values for titanium plates were somewhat greater than for stainless plates. Comparative results for titanium versus stainless specialty plates indicated that dimensions rather than modulus of elasticity was the primary factor effecting equivalent bending stiffness in the elastic region.

CONCLUSIONS

1. ISO 9585 test method is useful for evaluating the bending properties of small specialized bone plates.

2. Moment of inertia rather than modulus of elasticity can have a greater influence on the equivalent bending stiffness of bone plates in the elastic region.

3. Bone plate length, cylindrical roller dimensions, flatness deviations, and plate orientation must be controlled for consistent bend test results.

REFERENCES

[1]   ISO 9585 Implants for Surgery - Method for Testing Bending Strengths and Stiffness of Bone Plates, International Organization for Standardization, 1988.

R. R. Peterson, G. E. Lynch, T. W. Brasher[1]

CYCLIC CANTILEVER FATIGUE TESTING OF
COMPRESSION HIP SCREW PLATES

REFERENCE: Peterson, R. R., Lynch, G. E., and Brasher, T. W., "Cyclic Cantilever Fatigue Testing of Compression Hip Screw Plates," Clinical and Laboratory Performance of Bone Plates, ASTM STP 1217, J. P. Harvey, Jr., and R. F. Games, Eds., American Society for Testing and Materials, Philadelphia, 1994.

ABSTRACT:

In order to evaluate the fatigue strength and fracture mode of various compression hip screw plates, five different hip screw plate designs manufactured by four different companies were evaluated by cantilever loading the lag screw in the horizontal position with a predetermined load until failure. The plate portion of the device was secured to force the fracture to occur in the lag screw, barrel, or barrel/plate junction. The different products exhibited three different fracture modes and displayed as much as a 25X difference in the fatigue life averages. Design, material and processing differences were cited for this wide range of fatigue performance. The load which was used was extremely severe and was designed to determine a finite life for each design under specific test conditions. This information could be used for comparison purposes and for standardizing future testing.

KEY WORDS:

compression, hip plates, fatigue, cantilever apex, lag screw

INTRODUCTION:

For the past 25 years, compression hip screw plates have been used to reduce and stabilize troublesome hip fractures. During this time, improvements have been made in both materials and designs resulting in stronger devices. Although full weightbearing prior to complete bony union is contraindicated, these devices are often subjected to high cyclic loading. Therefore, component fatigue strength becomes an issue.

PURPOSE:

The purpose of this study was to determine the fatigue life and mode of fracture of five currently available compression hip screw plate systems under specific test conditions.

[1] Associates of Smith & Nephew Richards Inc., Memphis, Tennessee, USA

MATERIALS AND METHODS:

Five different compression hip screw plates manufactured by four different companies were collected for testing, along with their respective lag screws and compressing screws. All plates were of 135° angle. If the system offered a choice of keyed or keyless, the samples were tested with the locking mechanism (i.e., pin, clip) in place. A minimum of five samples from each manufacturer were tested; however, dependent on availability up to 19 samples were tested.

Samples were placed in a specially designed test fixture to allow for pure cantilever loading. Anatomical positioning of the plate (20° off vertical axis) was not feasible for this test because, in the absence of bone stock, the lag screw would slide into the barrel upon initial loading. It was the scope of this study to force fracture in the lag screw, barrel, or barrel/plate junction (apex) area to mimic intertrochanteric and femoral neck fractures.

Figure 1 is a diagram of the holding fixture and demonstrates how the maximum load was determined. F_1 represents the direction of force applied to the hip screw system when positioned anatomically correct. While this load is 4.7 times body weight, it is a load which produced failures in a reasonable amount of time. When the loading direction is shifted to F_2 as desired for this test, the equivalent resultant moment ($M_1 = M_2$) is obtained at the barrel and apex when force F_2 is approximately 1334 Newtons (300 pounds). During the tests, load was applied from 133 Newtons (30 pounds) to 1334 Newtons (300 pounds) resulting in a most severe loading condition. A fatigue rate of three cycles per second was used in all tests.

Calculations for Figure 1

4.73 x Bodyweight = F_1 = 3158 Newtons (710 lbs)
M_1 = (44.45 mm) (F_2)
M_2 = (44.45 Sin 25°) (F_1)
M_1 = M_2
F_2 = (Sin 25°) (3158 Newtons)
F_2 = 1334 Newtons (300 lbs)

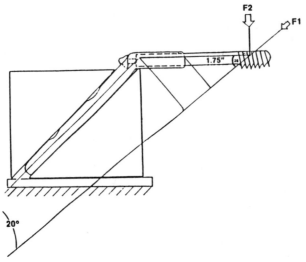

Figure 1 – Diagram of Test Setup

Loading was applied to the lag screw via a plunger with a roller. The point of roller contact was 82.5 mm (3-1/4") from the top of the barrel at the plate junction. The large buttress threads were machined off the top of each lag screw if necessary to assure exact location of the plunger.

A compressing screw was used in all tests to prevent the lag screws from migrating out. The constantly applied load kept the lag screws from migrating into the barrel. The distance that the lag screw was inserted into the barrel was kept constant such that the distance between the lag screw and the head of the compressing screw was 5 mm.

Figures 2 and 3 illustrate the different views of the actual test fixturing setup.

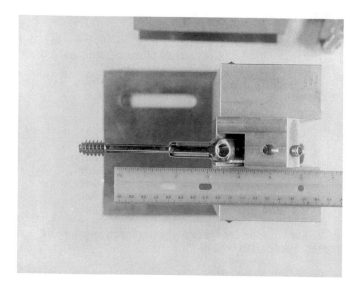

Figure 2 - Test setup (top view)

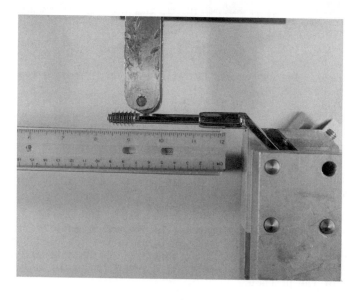

Figure 3 - Test Setup (Side View)

RESULTS AND DISCUSSION:

The fatigue life of each compression hip screw system was determined by averaging the number of cycles to failure. The table in Figure 4 summarizes the test results:

Figure 4

Product	Average	Standard Deviation	No. of Samples	Primary Failure Mode
A	220,807	49,634	7	Barrel
B	98,728	19,211	6	Apex
C	91,629	22,912	19	Lag Screw
D	21,806	3,833	5	Apex
E	8,896	5,486	5	Apex

Figure 5 is a bar graph depicting the average number of cycles to failure for each system tested.

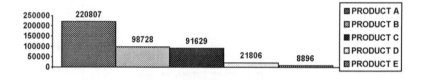

Figure 5 - Average cycles to failure for each product type.

In viewing the graph in Figure 5, it can be seen that Product A had the longest fatigue life. This can be attributed to the following three factors:

1.   Cold-forged 316L Stainless Steel Material,[1,2]
2.   Keyed design, and
3.   Glass-beaded surface finish[3]

The cold-forged material is very strong and, therefore, a longer fatigue life is expected as fatigue life is proportional to strength. The key design helps minimize stress risers in critical locations and also contributes to prolonged life. Finally, the glass-beaded surface finish imparts residual compressive stresses which again adds to the durability of the product.

Other products did not perform as well as Product A with Product E only obtaining 1/25 of Product A's fatigue life. Product E had a complicated design involving more machined and adjustable parts than conventional designs and when the extra notches of this design were combined with the notch sensitivity of the Titanium alloy it was made from, a lower fatigue strength was the result. In addition, the physical size of the implant with the material's lower modulus resulted in the implant deflecting much more than the other devices when the standardized load was applied. This higher strain will also reduce fatigue life.

Figure 6 illustrates the various features/locations of the compression hip screw plate.

While the failure mode/location of each product was not consistent, the primary failure mode was indicated in Figure 4. It can be seen that the most common failure mode is breakage at the apex by the compressing screw. This is a logical failure site due to the long bending moment at this location. The failure mode of Product A was in the barrel at the end of the lag screw. Elongation or wallowing of the barrel occurred until there was enough deflection to result in failure. The lag screw of Product C typically fractured transversely at the point it exited the barrel.

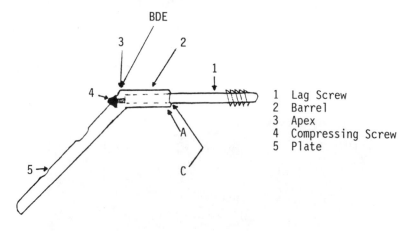

1	Lag Screw
2	Barrel
3	Apex
4	Compressing Screw
5	Plate

A	Typical failure location of Product A
B	Typical failure location of Product B
C	Typical failure location of Product C
D	Typical failure location of Product D
E	Typical failure location of Product E

Figure 6 – Failure locations

A lag screw failure, typical of Product C, may be seen in Figure 7.

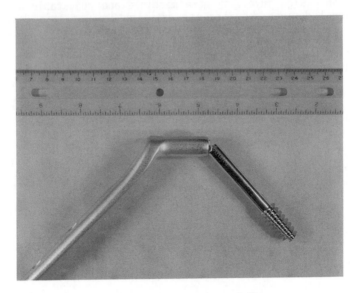

Figure 7 - Lag screw failure

A close-up of the failure location may be seen in Figure 8.

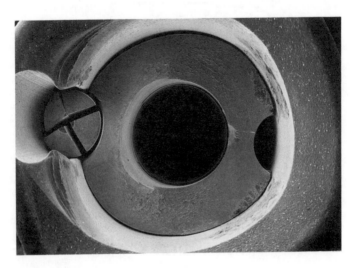

Figure 8 - SEM close-up of typical lag screw failure

Figure 9 displays a typical apex failure. Note the multiple crack
initiation sites in Figure 10.

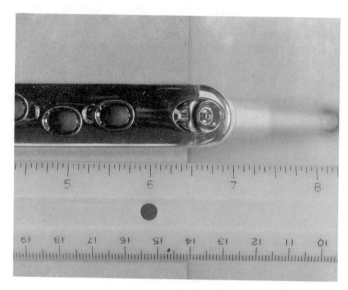

Figure 9 - Typical apex failure

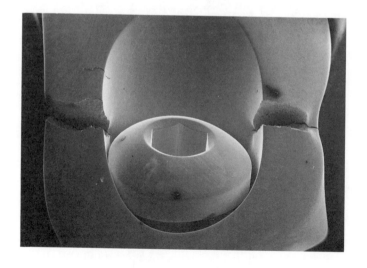

Figure 10 - SEM close-up of an apex failure

It should be noted that this study addressed the fatigue performance of the lag screw/barrel area of each system tested. Previous studies[4] report this area to be the most highly stressed area of intertrochanteric and femoral neck fractures. In this test scenario, support was supplied up to the apex of each system so that fracture in the plate area around the screw holes was not possible.

CONCLUSION:

This experiment was extremely severe and was designed to determine a finite life for the systems tested under specific test conditions, and provides comparative fatigue values of the various devices tested. Such a test method might also be valuable in standardizing tests for future use.

REFERENCES

1. Bardos, D. I., Baswell, I., Garner, S., and Wigginton, R., "The Development of a New High Strength, Cold Forged 316 LVM Stainless Steel," Trans. Soc. Biomaterials, 1984.

2. Davidson, J. A. and Bardos, D. I., "Historical Need for High-Strength Biomedical Implant Materials," American Soc. Metals, WESTEC '85, March 1985, Technical Paper No. 8501-001.

3. Shetty, R. H., Gilbertson, L. N. and Jacobs, C. H., "The New Surface Finish--A Method of Improving the Properties of 316L Stainless Steel," Trans. Soc. Biomaterials, 1987.

4. Doppelt, S. H., "The Sliding Compression Screw--Today's Best Answer for Stabilization of Intertrochanteric Hip Fractures," Orthop. Clin. North Am., 1980, 11 (3) 607-622.

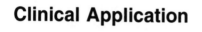

Clinical Application

Sadatoshi Kato,[1] Loren L. Latta, [1] and Theodore Malinin,[1]

THE WEAKEST LINK IN THE BONE - PLATE - FRACTURE SYSTEM; CHANGES WITH TIME

REFERENCE: Kato, S., Latta, L. L., and Malinin, T., "The Weakest Link in the Bone - Plate - Fracture System; Changes with Time," Clinical and Laboratory Performance of Bone Plates, ASTM STP 1217, J. P. Harvey, Jr. and R. F. Games, Eds., American Society for Testing and Materials, Philadelphia, 1994.

ABSTRACT: A retrospective analysis of data from a series of animal studies using the same animal model and methods of evaluation along with one prospective series of animals, provided comparable data on 83 dogs from 0 to 24 weeks post fracture. Closed diaphyseal fractures of the radius were created in 83 adult mongrel dogs. Forty-five were plated with 6 hole DCP stainless steel compression plates and 38 were plated with freeze-dried allograft bone plates. Mechanical evaluation of the strength of the healing bones was carried out at 0, 2, 4, 6, 12, and 24 weeks post fracture and analysis of the mode of failure, the location of failure and correlation with the strength of failure and time post fracture were evaluated for each different type of fixation. Both, the stainless steel and alloplated groups were divided into two subgroups: 1) refracture was carried out after removal of the fixation screws, and 2) refracture was carried out with the plates and screws intact. In the stainless steel plated animals at refracture, if the plates were removed: up to 4 weeks post injury, 100% of the refractures occurred through the fracture site (0% through screw holes); at 8 weeks, 50% (and 50%); at 12 weeks, 0% (and 100%); at 24 weeks, 75% (and 25%). In the stainless steel plated group where the plates were left intact at refracture, most of the refractures occurred at screw holes within the first 8 weeks postfracture, and by 24 weeks, the plates bent but remained attached to the bone, crushing the fracture site. In alloplated bones after screw removal, the refractures occurred at the fracture site consistently over the first 4 weeks; through screw holes at 8 weeks; and with mixed results at 12 and 24 weeks. If the screws were left intact at refracture in the alloplated group, 100% of the refractures occurred through the fracture site at 0 weeks, but from 8 weeks on, refractures were mixed In the stainless steel plated groups, whether the plate was left intact or whether the screws were removed, the refracture strength at screw holes never exceeded 50% of the original strength of the bone.

KEYWORDS: Fracture healing, fracture fixation, internal fixation, biomechanics

---
[1] Orthop. Surgeon & Research Fellow, Prof. & Dir. of Research, and Prof. , Assoc. Chairman for Academic Affairs & Dir. Tissue Bank, respectively; Univ. of Miami, Dept. Orthop. & Rehab., Box 016960, Miami, FL 33101

In the alloplated groups, after the bone had incorporated and the screws were no longer mechanically holding the plate in place, the refracture strengths were greater than 50% of the original strength of the bone, and when screws were left intact the screw hole strengths were greater than if the screws had been removed. Thus, this study shows that the fracture site appears to be at least as strong as the adjacent screw hole sites from about 8 weeks on in the plated dogs' radius, and the stress concentration effect at the screw hole sites remains whether the screws are intact or whether they have been removed when the screws are mechanically holding the plate in place up to 24 weeks post fracture.

INTRODUCTION:

Internal fixation with compression plates has proven to be an effective mean of dealing with unstable diaphyseal fractures. However, many clinical problems have surfaced even when optimum patient selection and surgical techniques are used. Refracture rates with plates intact and after plate removal are reported from 4% to 40% in long term studies [2,4]. Stress protection leading to osteoporosis[12], stress concentration from screw holes[1], retardation of healing[7,10] and disruption of blood supply[5] have all been blamed to varying degrees. Attempts at resolving these problems, include the reduction of stripping of the blood supply[5], use of less rigid plates[3,6,8,13,14], late[5] or early[14] plate removal, use of resorbable plates[6,8], fixation of plates without screws[9], etc. When the authors observed refracture of the fracture site after plate removal, as late as 2 years post fracture, the question arose as to when fracture site and the screw holes, and the bone strength beneath the plate were most vulnerable. The aim of the following study was to evaluate some of these mechanical parameters as a function of time postfracture to aid the surgeon in dealing with each problem in the proper sequence.

HYPOTHYSIS:

Based upon previous studies of isolated screws in the canine diaphysis[1], the authors hypothysize that the screw holes in the plated radius will weaken the bone to less than half its original strength after plate removal of a plated diaphyseal fracture. Based upon previous studies in the canine radius[12], the authors hypothysize that when the consturct reaches its peak strength (about 8 weeks post plating) the strength of the fracture site will reach the strength of the surrounding bone. In other words after plate removal, the fracture site strength will surpass the strength of the bone at the screw holes at 8 weeks or greater post plating.

METHODS:

A retrospective analysis of data from a series of animal studies, all using the same animal model and methods of evaluation along with the prospective series of animals provided comparative data on 83 dogs from 0 to 24 weeks post fracture[6,11]. All 83 adult mongrel dogs had minimally displaced (less than one cortical width) bending fractures of the radius and ulna created by a hydraulically controlled three-point bending device. Care was taken to obtain consistency of these simple transverse fractures in the midshaft area with the same degree of angular displacement to assure similar degrees of soft tissue damage for each injury. Seventy-one of these dogs were taken immediately post-fracture while under anesthesia to the surgical suite where an open reduction and internal fixation

Consistently from 2 weeks to 8 weeks, all of the refractures occurred through adjacent screw holes despite the fact that the maximum moment applied through the construct was at the fracture site. At 12 weeks postfracture 25% failed at the fracture site whereas 75% still failed through the adjacent screw holes. But at 24 weeks postfracture, all of the plates bent, the fracture site crushed, and no fractures occurred through adjacent screw holes. Thus, there was no complete mechanical failure or separation of the bone or bone plate construct throughout the testing at 24 weeks postfracture, but all bone-plate constructs were permanently angulated after testing.

TABLE I I - REFRACTURE STRENGTHS AT EACH SITE
Mechanical Healing in percent of control bone strength

GROUP	WKS POST FX	ULT. MOMENT MAX. ON BONE MEAN ± SD	PLATED FX SITE MEAN ± SD	/ % OF ALL	CONTROL SCREW HOLES MEAN ± SD	in % % OF ALL
SS	2	.18 ± .13	.18 ± .13	100	-----	0
PLATES	4	.23 ± .07	.23 ± .07	100	----	0
REMOVED	8	.44 ± .23	.32 ± .01	50	.42 ± .11	50
	12	.42 ± .12	----	0	.30 ± .08	100
	24	.56 ± .14	.48 ± .10	75	.43 ± ---	25
	0	1.14 ± .20	1.38 ± ---	17	.42 ± .02	83
SS	2	1.40 ± .23	----	0	.46 ± .03	100
PLATES	4	1.32 ± .15	----	0	.45 ± .02	100
INTACT	8	1.60 ± .42	----	0	.48 ± .05	100
	12	1.30 ± .28	.98 ± ---	25	.46 ± .03	75
	24	1.29 ± .18	1.29 ± .18	100	----	0
ALLO-	2	.21 ± .19	.21 ± .19	100	----	0
PLATES	4	.32 ± .08	.32 ± .08	100	----	0
NO	8	.73 ± .15	----	0	.62 ± .01	100
SCREWS	12	.77 ± .13	.93 ± ---	25	.50 ± .05	75
	24	.90 ± .10	.82 ± .04	50	.64 ± .02	50
ALLO-	0	.32 ± .04	.21 ± .03	100	----	0
PLATES	8	1.04 ± .16	.87 ± ---	25	.71 ± .99	75
WITH	12	1.16 ± .04	1.14 ± .03	75	.78 ± ---	25
SCREWS	24	1.08 ± .06	1.06 ± .08	100	----	0

was carried out; 12 were sacrificed prior to fracture so the procedure was evaluated immediately after injury.

Forty-five of the animals were plated with 3.5 mm, 6-hole stainless steel DCP compression plates. Thirty-eight of the animals were plated with reconstituted freeze-dried cortical bone plates fashioned from canine femurs. All animals were allowed weight bearing as tolerated in a cage environment with post operative antibiotics for the first 4 weeks. Animals which were kept for 8 weeks or more were placed in a long term carefacility with a more open environment which encouraged functional activity. Animals

TABLE I - DISTRIBUTION OF ANIMALS
Number of Animals/group

Type of plate V	Weeks post Fx >	0	2	4	8	12	24
	Refx with plates V						
Stainless Plates	Intact	6	4	4	4	4	4
(46 Dogs)	Removed	0	4	4	4	4	4
Allograft Plates	Intact	6	0	0	4	4	3
(37 Dogs)	Removed	0	4	4	4	4	4
Total (83 Dogs)		12	12	12	16	16	15

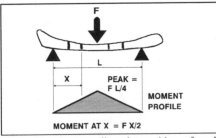

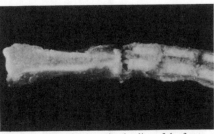

Figure 1 - By recording the position of each specimen in the loading apparatus, the moment at the location of the refracture could be calculated.

Figure 2 - The refracture site, healing of the fracture and effects of the plate on the underlying bone were evaluated from sagittal sections.

were sacrificed at 2, 4, 8, 12, and 24 weeks postfracture (in most groups)[*]. Twelve animals that were being sacrificed for other reasons, but had no pathologic conditions in

---

[*] The exceptions were for the allograft group with screws intact, the 2 week and 4 week groups were excluded because from the plate removal series it was evident that the allograft plate would not incorporate significantly until 8 weeks postfracture to contribute to the refracture strength of these bones. Therefore, there was no reason to believe that the refracture strength of the alloplated group should change from 0 to 4 weeks post fracture. Therefore, animals were sacrificed only at 0, 8, 12, and 24 weeks in this group.

their fore limbs, had their forearms fractured and right and left radii harvested. In 6 animals, one side was plated with the 3.5 mm. 6 hole stainless steel compression plate and refractured immediately with the plates and screws intact and the contralateral bone was fractured as control. In the other 6 animals, the radii on one side were plated with reconstituted freeze-dried cortical bone plates and were refractured in three-point bending along with the contralateral radii, Table I.

In all refracture comparisons, the injured limb, as well as the uninjured limb, were dissected post-mortem and the matched pair of radii recovered. Three point dorsal apex bending to failure was performed on each pair of radii and the stiffness, yield point and ultimate load at failure were recorded. Identification of the location of refracture and measurements of that location relative to the support and loading points in the three-point bending apparatus were noticed for each failure. Thus, the moment at the failure point could be calculated for each failure site, regardless of its location to the maximum bending moment point in the center of the three-point bending setup. The calculation of the moment at the failure point is shown in Figure 1. After refracture, all stainless steel parts were removed from all specimens. Specimens were x-rayed and then cut longitudinally through the medullary canal and carefully photographed for macroscopic observation, Figure 2. The region near the failure site and at the fracture site were then dissected free and decalcified for histologic evaluation.

RESULTS:

The ultimate moment for each failure site is reported in Table II along with the peak moment on the specimen and the structural stiffness of the specimen are reported in Table I. These values represent the maximum moment in the three-point bend set-up with load applied at the fracture site in each of the fractured bones and at a mirror image site of each of the unfractured bones. All values are reported in percent of control which is a ratio of the moment values in the experimental bones, divided by the identical values for the control side bone in the same animal, multiplied by 100, to give percent. In Table I, evaluation of the failure site is given in terms of the ultimate moment values at the failure site for those failures which occurred at the fracture site compared to ultimate moments values for failures which occurred through screw holes. The first column of values gives the ultimate moment at the fracture site (where the maximum moment was applied to the bone) at the time when failure occurred.

In the stainless steel plated group which had plates removed, the failure occurred through the fracture site consistently at 2 weeks and 4 weeks postfracture. At 8 weeks post-fracture, half of the failures occurred through the fracture site and half through adjacent screw hole sites. By 12 weeks postfracture, 100% of the failures occurred through adjacent screw hole sites, but by 24 weeks postfracture, a mixture of failures occurred; 75% through the original fracture site, 25% at adjacent screw holes. In the stainless steel plated groups tested with plates and screws intact (note that for this mode of loading the plate was on the tension band side of the bend test), the experimental sides were consistently stronger than the control side, (much different from those experimental bones tested after plate and screw removal). Immediately after plating, only 1 of 6 bones refractured through the fracture site and 5 refractured through an adjacent screw hole.

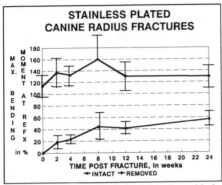

Figure 3a - Refracture strength in bending with the plate on the tension side compared to removed.

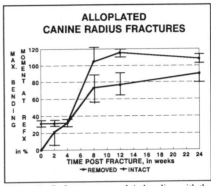

Figure 3b - Refracture strength in bending with the alloplate on the tension side compred to removed.

In the alloplated group, after screw removals, at 2 weeks and 4 weeks postfracture, the alloplate easily separated from the bone during the testing and apparently contributed very little to the strength of the construct. Refracture consistently occurred through the original fracture site. By 8 weeks postfracture, the alloplate had incorporated sufficiently into the cortical bone to provide substantial support and refracture occurred consistently through the adjacent screw holes. At 12 weeks postfracture, 25% of the refractures occurred through the original fracture site and 75% through the adjacent screw hole. At 24 weeks postfracture, the mixture of failure was 50-50 between fracture site and screw hole refractures. By 8 weeks postfracture, 25% of the failures occurred through the fracture site and 75% through adjacent screw holes. By 12 weeks postfractured, the situation had reversed and 25% of the refractures occurred through adjacent screw holes and 75% through the original fracture site. At 24 weeks postfracture, all refractures occurred through the original fracture site.

The overall bone-plate-fracture system steadily increased in strength up to 8 weeks postfracture in both stainless steel

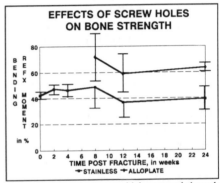

Figure 4 - For refractures which occurred through screw holes, the screws in alloplates weakened the bone less than those in stainless plate.

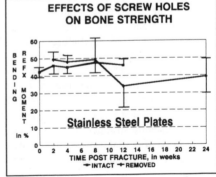

Figure 5a - The bending refracture strengths were essentially the same for intact or removed screws.

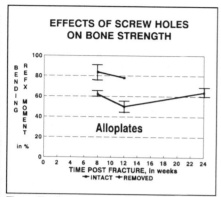

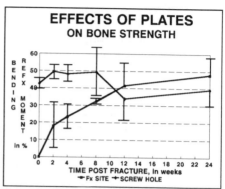

Figure 5b - Screw removal did seem to effect the bending refracture strength in alloplated bones.

Figure 6 - The bending refracture strength at the fracture site reached that of the screw holes at 8-12 weeks post fracture.

plated groups, see Fig. 3a. This trend leveled-off at 12, weeks and 24 weeks with no statistically significant changes from 8 weeks on. The alloplated bones continued a steady rise in strength with time showing a statistically significant increase from 8 weeks to 24 weeks, see Fig. 3b. Like the stainless steel plated group with plates and screws intact, the alloplate group with plates and screws intact, rose steadily to 8 weeks, leveled-off, and had no statistically significant changes from 8 weeks on. There was a statistically significant increase in the screw hole strength measured where refracture occurred through a screw hole in the alloplated group compared to the stainless steel plated groups, see Fig. 4. The fracture site strength was significantly stronger after plate removal at 24 weeks in the alloplated group versus the stainless steel plated bones. The stainless steel plated bones, when tested with the plates intact were significantly stronger than the alloplated bones at 0 and 8 weeks postfracture. There was no difference at any time period in the strength at screw holes of the stainless steel plated group regardless of whether the screws were left intact or removed, see Fig. 5a. Only at 12 weeks was there a statistically significant difference between the bending strength of the screw holes which failed with the screws intact compared to those removed (P < .01, by student's t-test). After screw removal, the screw holes in the alloplated bones were significantly stronger in bending than those in the stainless steel plated bones at 8 and 12 weeks (P < .05 and .01 by student's t-test), which were the only weeks where enough samples were available for statisical comparison, Fig. 5b.

Although the refracture strengths through the screw holes did not improve with time, the refracture strengths of the original fracture site did, see Fig. 6. The fracture site strength in bending was significantly less than the screw hole strengths only at 2 and 4 weeks (P < .005 by student's t-test), then seemed to reach the bending strength at the screw holes between 8 and 12 weeks.

DISCUSSION:

Study Design and Comparison to other Animal Studies

Three-point bending is not the ideal design to test the weakest part of the system since it applies a higher moment at one particular region than it does at another region and in this instance both of those regions were under evaluation. This, however, is a retrospective review of information that was collected from studies which were originally designed to evaluate the strength at the fracture site. Although this model did not work well for the original study (because many refractures occurred through screw holes), the data was consistent enough to provide some interesting insight into some questions which were not intended to be addressed by the original study design. Although it would be ideal to redo 90 dogs in 4.0 bending or in torsion so that a uniform moment would be created across a region of screw holes, as well as fracture site, this is impractical to do particularly when the data that is available is sufficient to evaluate these differences. Thus, in the evaluation of this data, the information on the incidence of refracture at the fracture site compared to incidence of refractures through screw hole is probably not as important as the actual refracture moments at those failure sites.

Clinically, refractures occur in both bending and torsion and can occur from a direct blow which would induce a maximum moment at a particular site in the bone similar to the testing techniques utilized in these studies. However, in a torsional refracture, or a refracture in bending induced by an eccentric axial load from functional activity, one would expect a more uniform moment along the bone and the site of refracture would be more predictable from the numbers given from this study in refracture ultimate moment rather than incidence of refracture for the three-point bend test. The numbers, however, are quite useful and produce some interesting results of clinical relevance.

After plate removal with stainless steel plated bones, even at 6 months postfracture in the dog (which is probably equivalent to 9 months or more in the human in a similar forearm bone), the refracture strength at the fracture site was not significantly less than the fracture site strength at 8 weeks postfracture but it was less than 50% of the original strength of the bone. In studies up to 12 weeks post fracture, the peak strength of the bone was at 8 weeks and the bone appeared to be getting weaker after 8 weeks[6,12]. Cortical thinning[12] may contribute to weakening of both the fracture site and the screw holes, see Fig. 7, and the effective cortical thickening of the healed alloplate may

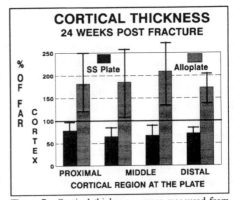

Figure 7 - Cortical thicknesses were measured from the saggittal cuts in the gross view (Fig. 2).

have contributed to the increased strength of the alloplated bones or the apparent recovery from stress concentration at the screw holes, see Fig. 7. Cortical thinning led Uhthoff[13] to experiment with early plate removal to try to prevent the loss in bone strength after 8 weeks in the dog.

In this study, the refracture strength at the screw holes never reached above 50% of the original strength of the bone whether the screws were removed or intact at anytime postfracture. This does not mean that all of the screw hole sites were less than 50% of the strength of the original intact bone, because many of the screw hole sites did not experience failure and so their failure moment was not measured. However, in those screw holes which appear to be the weakest, and a refracture did occur, their failure consistently was under 50% of the original strength of the bone.

In previous work by Burstein[1] in similar animal bones, it was noticed that a single screw placed in the bone, not attached to a plate or other load bearing device, with no fracture in the bone, would cause only a temporary stress concentration effect and would lower the bone below 50% of its original strength for only a very short duration. Remodeling around that screw would bring the bone back to its original strength within about 16 weeks after application. If the screws were removed after 16 weeks and the bone refractured, the stress concentration effect would be reactivated and the bone would become approximately 50% of its original strength. This, however, would recover rapidly within a matter of a few weeks and the bone would regain its original strength. Comparing that study to the present study it appears that this phenomenon is only true for screws which are passively placed in the bone and not attached to a load bearing device. The most similar circumstance to that in this study would be with the alloplated screws at 8 weeks or more postfracture, since these screws were no longer the load bearing attachments for the plate to the bone. The bone had incorporated into the original cortical bone to such an extent that the screws were effectively passive screws at some point beyond 8 weeks post fracture. In these instances, note that the refracture strength at those screw hole sites were significantly greater than the refracture strength noted in the stainless steel plated bones.

Potential Clinical Relevance

The potential clinical significance of this work is the strong evidence to indicate that whether one removes a stainless steel plate or leaves the plate intact, one can expect that the stress concentration effect of the screw hole sites for those screws attached to the plate will remain significant for extended periods of time. Conversely, isolated lag screws independent of the plate are probably not continued sources of stress concentration (similar to the studies of Burstein[1]). The only indication from this study that remodeling may eventually strengthen those screw hole sites is that refractures did not occur in those screw hole sites at moments near to the original strength of the bone at 24 weeks postfracture when the plates and screws were left intact. Thus, this work supports the rationale for early removal of plates and for post operative protection after plate removal. This work also supports the idea that isolated lag screws, not attached to a plate, may be left alone without need for long term protection.

ACKNOWLEDGEMENTS:

The authors acknowledge the contributions of the following people (in alphabetical order) on the earlier phases of this work: Ralph Alvarez, John Cohen, Donald Mullis, Frank Reyes, Augusto Sarmiento. Partial support by: University of Miami Biomechanics Laboratory at Mount Sinai Medical Center.

REFERENCES:

[1]   Burstein, AH, et.al.: Bone strength, J Bone Joint Surg, Vol. 54A, 1972, p. 1143.

[2]   Chrisman, OD, Snook, GA, "The problem of refracture of the tibia", Clin Orthop, Vol. 60, 1982, p. 217.

[3]   Harris, W, et.al., "Observation on fracture healing the mode of action of compression plates", J Bone Joint Surg, Vol. 55B, 1973, p. 214.

[4]   Hidaka, S. and Gustillo, R.B., "Refracture of bones of the forearm after plate removal", J Bone Joint Surg, Vol. 66A, 1984, p. 1241.

[5]   Jacobs, R, Rahn, B, Perren, S, "Effect of plates on cortical bone perfusion", Trans 26th Orthop Res Soc, Vol. 5, 1980, p.157.

[6]   Malinin, TI, et.al., "Healing of freeze-dried bone plates - comparison with compression plates", Clin Orthop, Vol. 190, 1984, p.281.

[7]   Olerud, S, Dankwardt-Lilliestrom, G, "Fracture healing in compression osteosynthesis", Acta Orthop Scand Suppl, #137, 1971.

[8]   Parsons, J, et.al., "Development of a variable stiffness, absorbable bone plate", Trans 25th Orthop Res Soc, Vol. 4, 1979, p. 168.

[9]   Partridge, AJ, "Nylon cerclage fixation for osteoporotic fractures", J Bone Joint Surg, Vol. 62B, 1980, p. 123.

[10]   Perren, S, et al., "Cortical bone healing", Acta Orthop Scand Suppl, #125, 1969.

[11]   Sarmiento, A, Mullis, D, Latta, L, Alvarez, R, "A quantitative comparative analysis of fracture healing under the influence of compression plating vs. closed weight-bearing treatment", Clin Orthop, Vol. 149, 1980, p.232.

[12]   Uhthoff, HK, Dubuc, FL, "Bone structure in the dog under rigid internal fixation", Clin Orthop, Vol. 81, 1971, p. 165.

[13]   Uhthoff, HK, "The use of titanium -6L-4V plates in the treatment of fractures", Trans 24th Orthop Res Soc, Vol. 3, 1978, p.29.

[14]   Woo, S, Lonthriger, K, Akeson, W, et.al., "Less rigid internal fixation plates: historical perspectives and new concepts", J Orthop Res, Vol. 1, 1983, pp. 431-449.

Ann Ouellette[1], Sadatoshi Kato[2], Katsumi Nakamura[2], Loren L. Latta[3], William E. Burkhalter[4]

MECHANICAL EVALUATION OF INTERNAL AND EXTERNAL FIXATION FOR METACARPAL FRACTURES

REFERENCE: Ouellette, A., Kato, S., Nakamura, K., Latta. L. L., and Burkhalter, W. E., **"Mechanical Evaluation of Internal and External Fixation for Metacarpal Fractures,"** Clinical and Laboratory Performance of Bone Plates, ASTM STP 1217, J. P. Harvey, Jr., and R. F. Games, Eds., Amercian Society for Testing and Materials, Philadelphia, 1994.

ABSTRACT: The purpose of this study was to compare fixation techniques for metacarpal fractures under the most and least mechanically demanding situations: bone contact and no bone contact and to test the potential role of soft tissues in providing a mechanically significant tension band to support the fixation. Two hundred fifty-eight (258) human metacarpals fixed in formalin (some dissected free of soft tissue and others in intact hands) were mechanically tested in 3 point, apex dorsal bending with midshaft transverse osteotomies to compare five (5) types of internal fixation and nine configurations of external fixation. In addition, eighty-four (84) proximal phalanges were fixed with both dorsal and lateral plates and tested in 3 point bending with and without soft tissue support. Reduction with end to end contact was obtained in the first series and a 3 mm. gap at the osteotomy site was obtained in a second series. The dorsal plate provided the greatest rigidity and strength with bone contact. External fixation was at least as strong and rigid as wire internal fixation. All configurations of external fixation were were stronger and more rigid than internal fixation with a gap at the fracture site. Double frame configurations were statistically significantly more rigid and stronger than single frames in almost all configurations tested and pin placement nearest the A-P plane were the most rigid and the strongest. More compliant fixation systems were supplemented the most in by intact soft tissues, but all fixation systems incrested in strength and stiffness with intact soft tissues. Lateral plates were comparable in strength and stiffness to dorsal plates in dorsal bending only when soft tissues were intact.

KEYWORDS: Fracture fixation, hand fractures, internal fixation, external fixation, biomechanics

INTRODUCTION: There are numerous methods of fixation to retain the reduction of diaphyseal fractures of the metacarpals. Numerically, most fractures of the metacarpals can be treated by the application of closed reduction and plaster fixation. However, certain unstable fractures need to be effectively immobilized by the use of Kirschner wires or alternatively by the use of the AO small fragment instrumentation. These techniques are widely employed for a variety of fresh fractures involving small tubular bones.

[1]Prof. & Chief Hand Surg. Service, Dept. Orthop. & Rehab., Univ. of Miami, PO Box 016960, Miami, FL 33101

[2]Orthop. Surgeon, Research Fellow, Dept. Orthop. & Rehab., Univ. of Miami, PO Box 016960, Miami, FL 33101

[3]Prof. & Dir. of Research, Dept. Orthop. & Rehab., Univ. of Miami, PO Box 016960, Miami, FL 33101

[4]Former Prof. & Assoc. Chairman for Medical Affairs, Dept. Orthop. & Rehab., Univ. of Miami, PO Box 016960, Miami, FL 33101, (Deceased)

On the other hand, fractures which have bone loss or extensive comminution cannot be stabilized with these standard internal fixation techniques. External fixation provides a potential means of handling these more difficult fractures. The skeletal stabilization should be biomechanically rigid enough to allow immediate finger joint mobility to avoid a loss of range of motion and joint stiffness often associated with immobilization[1,2,3,4,5]. Thus, the primary goal of treatment is to obtain early rigidity by fracture fixation.

Although numerous studies have defined the mechanical role of internal fixation in the hand[6,7,8], little is known about external fixation[9]. Knowledge of the mechanical advantages of each method would be very helpful to defining their indications.

The following study was designed to evaluate parameters of external fixation which best supports the most rugged mechanical demands on the metacarpals and to compare internal to external fixation methods and the potential support of soft tissues.

METHODS: Moistened human cadaveric metacarpals were chosen for testing, since the effect on bone strength of embalming was within the normal limit of variations from bone to bone[11]. The metacarpals had transverse osteotomies created at the midshaft area and subsequently underwent three point bending tests after fixation with the following techniques:

(1)   Dorsal plate, (DP), fixation with an AO small fragment plate fixed with four 2.7 mm. cortical screws with no interfragmentary screw applied (Fig. 1).

(2)   Crossed Kirschner wires, (KW), of 1.25 mm. diameter. (The test of these two internal fixation techniques was performed to compare our data with the previous study reported by Black et al. at the University of Utah Medical Center[3].

(3)   Intramedullary fixation devices,(IMFD), of the Lewis design were tested both with and without soft tissues. It was impossible to maintain bone contact without soft tissue tension over the metacarpal so all data on isolated bones was considered to be with a gap at the osteotomy site.

(4)   External fixation, (EF), utilizing a Hoffmann apparatus in three positions: With the plane of application of the pins in the sagittal plane, at a 45 degree angle oblique to the sagittal plane and in the frontal plane. (This defines the anticipated maximum, one intermediate and minimum rigidity for each of the configurations, respectively). Three configurations of the mini-Hoffmann were applied in each of these positions: (a) half pins and one side frame, (b) through pins and two side frames and (c) double half pins and double side frames.

(5)   External fixation utilizing a mini-Hoffmann vise clamp with double half-pin configuration with the planes of application of the pins at +45 degrees to the sagittal plane. The Hoffmann vise clamp was used with 1.5 mm. threaded pins.

Two separate internal fixation configurations and nine external fixation configurations were tested with cortical contact at the osteotomy site in one series of groups (Fig. 1a) and with a 3 mm. gap at the osteotomy site in a second series (Fig. 1b) with no soft tissues and compared to the same fixation of osteotomies in intact hands.

In the authors' experiences, most mechanical failures, clinically, result in dorsal angulation. Thus, mechanical testing was performed in three point

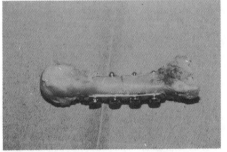

Figure 1a - One group of cadaveric metacarpal bones had mid-shaft, transverse osteotomies fixed with bone contact.

bending to complete failure of
each specimen as follows: Each
metacarpal was supported at the
proximal and the distal ends so
that the bone rested on the two
supports allowing complete freedom of rotation at the supports (Fig. 2). The supports
were 35.0 mm. apart and bending
was accomplished by pressing
down at the center of the specimen until bending was completed. The test proceeded to
failure of either the bone, the
fixation, or the device in the
following manner: The ram was
lowered onto the specimen at a
constant deflection rate of 1.0
mm. per second and a force tra-
nsducer was attached to the ram
so that a load could be monitored throughout the bending
test.

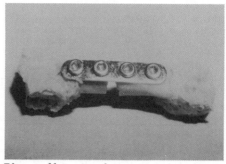

Figure 1b - Another group was fixed
with a 3 mm gap at the osteotomy
site.

The load and displacement were monitored throughout the test and
in each case a relatively linear portion of the graph was noted. Any
deviation from that linear portion of the graph was considered to be the
yield point of the test and the peak load reached during the test was
considered to be the ultimate load. For these yield and ultimate load
values, the yield and the ulti-
mate moments were calculated from
$M=PL/4$, where M is the moment, P
is the load applied at the midsp-
an and L is the span between the
two supports.

The area under the linear
portion of the graph was used to
calculate the energy to yield.
The bending stiffness was calculated from $PL^3/48d$, where P is the
applied load, L^3 is the moment, P
is the load applied at the midsp-
an and L is the span of the supports, and d is the deflection at
the mid span. Thus, P/d is the
slope of the linear portion
load/displacement curve.

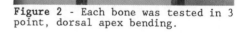

Figure 2 - Each bone was tested in 3
point, dorsal apex bending.

A total of two hundred and
sixteen (216) metacarpal bones
were mechanically tested with ap-
proximately nine specimens use in each of the 25 groups (Tables I & II),
without soft tissues and forty-two (42) in intact hands.

Based on the good comparison between our data and Black's[3] for the
crossed Kirschner wire fixed metacarpals without soft tissues, it was
felt that the external fixation measurements would also be comparable to
their measurements for intraosseous wire and Kirschner wire combination
fixation since the mechanism of failure and means of applying rigidity
to the bone is quite similar between these techniques of fixation (i.e.
the rigidity is more related to slipping of the pins or wires through
the holes in the bone or to the actual rigidity of the wires and pins
themselves and not related to mechanical failure of the bone material).
Thus, the data from Black[3] for internal fixation with bone contact is
included in Table I (with their permission) for comparison to internal
fixation values obtained in this study with a gap at the fracture site
and to external fixation values.

The stiffness and strength measurements and calculations were compared statistically by students' t-test with compensation for multiple group comparisons.

RESULTS: There was a very significant drop in the rigidity of the dorsal plate fixation prior to yield (which occurred only slightly before the gap had closed), with approximately a 4-fold decrease of rigidity (statistically significant by student's T test with P < .001).

TABLE I
INTERNAL FIXATION

CONFIGURATION	NO.	STRUCTURAL STIFFNESS EI in N·m²		YIELD MOMENT in N·m		ULTIMATE MOMENT in N·m		ANGULATION AT YIELD in DEGREES	
		AVE.	S.D.	AVE.	S.D.	AVE.	S.D.	AVE.	S.D.
DP + Lag Screw, Contact[1]	8	.56	.116	3.50	.88	5.59	2.01	6.3	2.3
DP, 4 hole, Contact[1]	8	.51	.211	4.00	2.44	6.22	3.91	5.7	1.8
DP, 4 hole, Contact	13	.33	.067	3.24	.76	3.43	.68	5.4	1.4
DP, 4 hole, Gap	9	.08	.023	.70	.23	2.83	.67	5.9	1.7
DP, Intact Hand, Gap	8	.11	.081			5.09	1.76		
Crossed KW, Contact[1]	8	.07	.032	.59	.25	.90	.40	11.1	3.9
Crossed KW, Contact	7	.06	.017	.73	.18	.96	.27	9.1	2.8
Crossed KW, Gap	5	.02	.001	.47	.09	.56	.06	17.6	13
Crossed KW Intact Hand, Gap	5	.64	.020			5.07	1.52		
IO Wire, Contact	8	.07	.055	.36	.14	.68	.33	5.6	3.9
IO Wire + K-Wire, Contact[1]	8	.06	.031	.43	.21	.80	.31	7.1	3.2
IMFD, Gap	17	.04	.076			.81	.41		
IMFD, Intact Hand, Gap	27	.05	.022			3.65	1.99		

S.D. - standard deviation
IO - interosseous

[1]Black D, Mann RA, Constine R, Daniels AU: "Comparison of Internal Fixation Techniques in Metacarpal Fractures". J Hand Surg 10A:466-72, 1985.

External fixation configurations tended to provide the greatest rigidity when the plane of the pins was aligned in the plane of bending, Table II.   A small reduction in rigidity was noted as the plane of the pins became oblique to the plane of the bending and the least rigid configuration was obtained when the plane of the pins was perpendicular to the plane of bending.   The only exception to this was with the double, half-pin configuration when a gap was created at the fracture site.   In this instance, the rigidity was greater when the pins were placed at an oblique angle to the plane of bending than when the pins were placed with one frame in the plane of bending and the other frame perpendicular to the plane of bending.   This difference in stiffness was not statistically significant, however.

In all instances, the rigidity of the fixation was reduced when a gap of 3 mm. was created at the fracture site, see Tables II.   The reduction in the stiffness caused by the creation of fracture site gap was not significant statistically in any of the external fixation configurations, however, except for the double, half-pin configuration using Hoffmann vise clamps.   In this instance, the reduction in stiffness was approximately 30% which was statistically significant in a student's T test with P < .05.

Comparing external fixation configurations, all double frame configurations were statistically significantly more rigid than single half-pin frames for each pin position tested with the following exception: The double thru-pin configuration at an oblique angle was not significantly stiffer than the single half-pin configuration at an oblique angle. These differences between single and double frame configurations were also statistically significant regardless of whether the bone ends were in contact or whether a gap existed at the fracture site. The Hoffmann vise clamps in the double half-pin configuration at an oblique angle to the plane of bending was significantly more rigid than any of the other configurations tested with and without a gap at the fracture site (Table II).

TABLE II
EXTERNAL FIXATION

CONFIGURATION	NO	STRUCTURAL STIFFNESS EI in N·m²		YIELD MOMENT in N·m		ULTIMATE MOMENT in N·m		ANGULATION AT YIELD in DEGREES	
		AVE.	S.D.	AVE.	S.D.	AVE.	S.D.	AVE.	S.D.
SHP, AP, Contact	8	.09	.013	1.11	.12	1.29	.12	8.7	1.3
SHP, AP, Gap	8	.07	.012	1.41	.33	1.65	.31	13.1	2.1
SHP, Oblique, Contact	8	.08	.025	1.38	.38	2.23	.39	11.4	3.4
SHP, Oblique, Gap	7	.08	.035	1.15	.22	1.83	.11	10.5	4.8
SHP, Oblique, Intact Hand	2	.10	.009			7.84	.74		
SHP, ML, Contact	8	.05	.009	.76	.21	1.52	.42	10.7	2.0
SHP, ML, Gap	8	.02	.004	.99	.15	1.08	.15	31.3	5.7
DHP, AP, Contact	12	.14	.029	2.07	.28	2.98	.64	10.3	2.2
DHP, AP, Gap	7	.13	.014	1.76	.09	2.32	.32	9.6	1.1
DHP, Oblique, Contact	8	.14	.040	1.70	.24	2.16	.17	8.6	2.5
DHP, Oblique, Gap	9	.15	.039	1.43	.26	2.51	.15	6.5	1.7
DTP, AP, Contact	9	.14	.045	2.11	.39	3.10	.61	10.2	3.2
DTP, AP, Gap	7	.11	.014	1.80	.38	2.57	.31	11.1	1.4
DTP, Oblique, Contact	12	.09	.017	1.55	.15	2.03	.41	12.0	2.3
DTP, Oblique, Gap	9	.09	.018	1.57	.33	2.82	.11	12.5	2.6
DTP, ML, Contact	8	.08	.016	1.40	.46	2.64	.29	12.6	2.6
DTP, ML, Gap	9	.08	.023	1.01	.21	2.21	.24	9.2	2.8
Vice Clamp, Obl., Contact	11	.34	.086	4.07	.85	4.51	.91	8.3	2.1
Vice Clamp, Oblique, Gap	10	.26	.101	2.92	1.22	4.09	1.16	7.8	3.1

S.D. - standard deviation
AP - pins applied in the anterior-posterior plane
ML - pins applied in the medial-lateral plane
Oblique - pins applied in a plane 45° oblique to the AP & ML planes
SHP - Single half-pin External Fixation
DHP - Double half-pin External Fixation
DTP - Double through-pin External Fixation

The ultimate moment in all types of fixation significantly increased with soft tissues intact, (P < .005), see Figure 3. The structural stiffness with non-rigid fixation (KW, EF, and IMFD) increased with intact soft tissues. DP fixation exhibited a much less dramatic change; < 80% in ultimate load, see Table I. With plates applied through a surgical wound, the rigid fixation behaved more like isolated metacarpals with a 3mm gap than those with bone contact. It was readily apparent that coaptation and compression was not achieved with these miniplates as one would expect with a dynamic compression plate in a major long bone and coaptation was apparently easier with isolated metacarpals.

For proximal phalanx fixation, there was a significant difference in strength and stiffness for dorsal plate location over lateral plate location, as expected, in isolated bones. However, in intact hands, there was no difference, Fig. 4.

DISCUSSION: The relative effect of the gap on plated bone stiffness in this study compares well with theoretical predictions based on strain measurements in fresh bone[9]. Thus, even though the plated bones did not behave as well as fresh plated bones mechanically, the relative effect of the gap on mechanical behavior was similar to fresh bone measurements.

The relative difference of values between the external fixators and pin and wire internal fixation techniques in this model are probably good comparisons because of the similarity in failure mechanism, which is similar to those failures observed clinically: slippage of the wires through the bone and bent wires. They also should reflect more closely the behavior anticipated in fresh bone because the rigidity and mechanism of failure is related to the elasticity and yielding of the fixation devices, not the bone. However, comparing these values to the plate fixation techniques is probably dubious as plate fixation in a few fresh

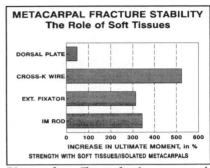

Figure 3 - The relative strength increase was more predominant in the more compliant forms of fixation.

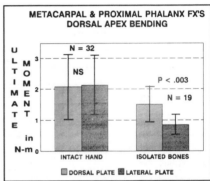

Figure 4 - Fixation strength was similar for dorsal and lateral plating when the soft tissues were left intact.

bones provided comparable rigidity, but much higher strength due to very different failure mechanisms.

The mechanisms of failure were very different for each fixation technique. Thus, ultimate moment measurements were inconsistent in the values and insignificance for comparing groups. The ultimate moment measurements were not comparable to the internal fixation groups for most of the external fixation configurations tested since there was no clear ultimate mechanical failure of the system for this particular mechanical test. The rigidity of the system primarily seemed to be controlled by the bending of the pins between the bone and clamps, and the twisting and sliding of the pins in the bone. In some instances, the bone would crack through a pinhole and a clear mechanical failure would result, but this end result was not consistent enough to provide reasonable ultimate moment data for comparison between groups.

For the internal fixation configurations, an ultimate failure was a significant piece of information as this usually was associated with splitting of the bone through a screw hole (in the case of the dorsal plate) or pullout of the crossed K-wires or splitting of the bone through a wire hole (in the case of wire fixation). The ultimate failure for each of the internal fixation configurations occurred at a relatively small degree of angulation. Thus, the ultimate moment data is potentially of clinical significance for internal fixation. The external fixation, however, had such a great range of elastic behavior that the ultimate, and sometimes the yield points were beyond what one might consider clinical failure. Thus, the angulation at yield may be more important than the yield or ultimate moments in many instances of evaluating this data relative to clinical failure criteria (Table I & II). Since no clinical criteria exists, to the knowledge of the authors, that identifies a value for acceptable stiffness of fixation or strength of fixation, this data can only be used in a relative sense to help identify the trends in control of fixation stiffness and strength that the surgeon controls using these methods.

Clinically, it is not practical to apply pins on the dorsal or lateral sides of the metacarpal. But mechanically those positions provide the maximum and minimum strength and stiffness behaviors for apex dorsal bending. Thus, these placements in this study represent the bounds of behavior of each fixation system and the maximum degree of control that the placement provides, mechanically. This is important information for the surgeon to weigh when deciding about the trade-offs between optimizing mechanics vs. the biological or clinical variables affected by the surgical procedure.

Soft tissues play a major role in providing mechanical stability and resilience with non-rigid forms of metacarpal fracture fixation. With plate fixation, although the rigidity is not the level achieved in major long bone fixation, the soft tissues are stressed much less and thus plate fixation is recommended in instances where protection of soft tissue injuries or repairs is needed. If a plate is necessary for fixation of a phalangeal fracture, then one can place it dorsally or laterally and achieve similar mechanical stability. By placing the plate laterally, there is less tendon involvement with potentially fewer adhesions thus leaving the extensor mechanism in a more functional state. Also, with an understanding of the importance of the soft tissues in the mechanical behavior of hand fractures, one can better evaluate those mechanical studies in the literature which ignore the role of soft tissues. For compliant forms of fixation, the effects of the soft tissues will probably be very significant.

ACKNOWLEDGEMENTS: Special thanks to Dr. Black and colleagues[3] for sharing their data, methods, and advice. This work was supported in part by Howmedica Inc. and performed in part at the University of Miami, Orthopaedics Biomechanics Laboratory at Mt. Sinai Medical Center, Miami Beach, Florida.

REFERENCES:
[1]   Alexander H, Langrana N, Massengill JB, Weiss AB: Development of new methods for phalangeal fracture fixation. J Biomech Vol. 14, 1981, pp 377-87

[2]   Belasole R: Physiological fixation of displaced and unstable fractures of the hand. Orthop Clin of N A, Vol. 11, No. 3, July 1980

[3]   Black D, Mann RA, Constine R, Daniels AU: Comparison of internal fixation techniques in metacarpal fractures. J Hand Surg Vol. 10A, 1985, pp 466-72

[4]   Fyfe IS, Mason S: The mechanical stability internal fixation of fractured phalanges. Hand Vol. 2, 1979, pp 50-58

[5]   Lister G: Intraosseous wiring of the digital skeleton. J Hand Surg Vol. 3, 1978, pp 427-35

[6]   Massengill JB, Alexander H, Parson JR, Schecter MJ: Mechanical analysis of Kirschner wire fixation in a phalangeal model. J Hand Surg Vol. 4, 1979, pp 351-6

[7]   Massengill JB, Alexander H, Langrana N, Mylod A: A phalangeal fracture model-quantitative analysis of rigidity and failure. J Hand Surg Vol. 7, 1982, pp 264-70

[8]   Muller ME, Allgower M, Schneider R, Wilenegger H: Manual of internal fixation, Springer-Verlag, Berlin, 1979, pp. 198.

[9]   Pawluk RJ et al.: Effects of bone gaps on internal fixation stability. Trans 28th Orthop. Res. Soc., Vol. 7, 1982, p 325

[10] Stuchin SA, Kummer FJ: Stiffness of small-bone external fixation method: an experimental study. J Hand Surg Vol. 9A, 1984, pp 718-724

[11] Swanson SA: Biomechanical characteristics of bone. Adv Biomed Eng Vol. 1, 1981, pp 137-187

[12] Viktor ME, Chiu DW, Beasley RW: The place of skeletal fixation in surgery of the hand. Clin in Plastic Surg, Vol. 8, No. 1, January, 1981

M. Rayhack, M.D.[1], Seth I. Gasser, M.D.[2], Edward L. Milne, BSc.[3], Loren L. Latta, Ph.D.[3]

MECHANICS OF ULNAR OSTEOTOMIES AND PLATE FIXATION

ERENCE: Rayhack, J. M., Gasser, S. I., Milne, E. L., and Latta, L., "Biomechanics of Ulnar Osteotomies and Plate Fixation," ical and Laboratory Performance of Bone Plates, ASTM STP 1217, Paul Harvey, Jr. and Robert F. Games, Eds., American Society for ing and Materials, Philadelphia, 1994.

STRACT: Osteotomies to shorten the ulna have proven to be an effective procedure for ar positive wrist syndrome. However, the procedure has been fraught with a number of chanical problems which have limited its clinical and biological success. This work poses a solution for some of these mechanical problems and tests this hypothesis in the oratory and the clinical setting.

Twenty pairs of human ulnas (5 pairs in each group) had shortening osteotomies formed. One side had conventional transverse, "free-hand" cuts, coaptation by hand and npression and neutralization by a standard A0 3.5 mm, 7-hole DCP Plate. The tralateral ulna had a fixture attached to the bone to control the cutting saw and the bone ments throughout the $45°$ osteotomy cuts and controlled coaptation and compression with an afragmentary lag screw and neutralization with a 2.5 mm, low profile, 7-hole plate. After the co-aptation, npression and neutralization were complete, the fixture was removed, and each ulna was elastically tested bending (in two planes) and torsion stiffness, and for strength in apex volar bending. Bending stiffness of h plate designs was also measured.

Structural stiffness was clearly greater in torsion testing for the oblique osteotomy at a significance l of $P < .04$. No biomechanical difference was identified in the AP and lateral bending tests despite the that the low profile plate was only half the bending rigidity of the standard plate.

In a clinical trial, twenty-three transverse osteotomies were compared to seventeen oblique otomies using the described instruments. The healing rate and consistency was improved for the oblique otomy group compared to the transverse osteotomy group by 10.9 versus 20.6 weeks to healing in 100% us 96% completely healed cases, respectively.

The osteotomy instrumentation system not only provided the surgeon with a means of reducing rative time, post-operative complications, ease of implementation and reduced hardware bulk in the cutaneous region, but also improved the mechanical and clinical performance for short and long term due he precision and configuration of the construct, requiring less mechanically demanding hardware.

YWORDS: Plate Fixation, Surgical instruments, Osteotomy

RODUCTION:

The ulnar shortening procedure was first introduced by Milch in 1941[9], however, plate fixation of the otomy was not described in the literature until 1974[1]. In this publication, Cantero introduced the iguing concept of the Z-cut osteotomy., In 1977, Cantero described the oblique osteotomy using a double technique.[2] Four subsequent articles[3,4,7,10] have described the clinical results of ulnar shortening otomies stabilized by an internal fixation plate.

rthopaedist, Wrist and Hand Center of Tampa, 4728 N,. Habana Drive, Tampa, FL 33614

rthopaedist, Sports Medicine, Florida Orthopaedic Institute, 4175 East Fowler Ave., Tampa, FL 33617

djunct Instructor & Professor, respectively, Department of Orthopaedics and Rehabilitation, D-27, versity of Miami, School of Medicine, Box 016960, Miami, FL 33101

Ulnar shortening osteotomies are used to provide relief of pain and return of grip strength in patients with ulnar positive wrists, a common problem after distal radius fracture, Essex-Lopresti injuries, Monteggia fractures, etc. The indications for ulnar shortening osteotomies have now broadened substant to include: triangular fibrocartilage tears, ulnar impaction syndrome[8], lunotriquetral tears, and incongrue of the distal radial-ulnar joint[7]. This suggests that, in the future, increasing number of osteotomy proced will be performed.

However, this procedure is not benign, is technically demanding, is associated with minor malalignment, prolonged healing time, high rate of nonunion, and skin closure problems over bulky hard in a subcutaneous region. "Struggles with fixing the osteotomy" have been previously documented[2]. In technique, once the osteotomy was complete, two free bone fragments existed and it was the task of the operating surgeon to apply the plate without rotation while concurrently trying to compress the bone end the transverse osteotomy. Even the suggestion of fixation of the plate to one fragment[3] once the osteoto was performed still leaves the surgeon with a formidable surgical task.

HYPOTHESIS:

If the precision of the osteotomy, its co-aptation and compression can be optimized, the rigidity the implant can be reduced without loosing any rigidity of fixation of the construct while reducing the bu the hardware, improving rate of healing, and reducing the potential for late ulnar weakening associated w stress protection.

METHODS:

Twenty right/left paired human ulnas were dissected from formalin fixed specimens. An oblique osteotomy fixture (Figure 1) was fixed to one ulna of each pair and the osteotomy was followed by fixation with a low profile (2.5 mm), prototype slotted plate, plus a standard 2.7 mm interfragmentary lag screw and six standard 3.5 mm cortical screws. The cutting fixture establishes the locations of the three proximal screws that will hold the plate, as well as one of the distal screws. This fixture controls the bone during the osteotomy. Next the plate is attached to the proximal fragment and the compression fixture applied to the plate and bone secured to the proximal fragment by the most distal of the proximal screws, and to the distal fragment by the most proximal of the distal screws. The screw which holds the fixture to the distal fragment, passes through a slot in the plate so that the bone can be slid beneath the plate to compress against the proximal fragment. After coaptation and compression are completed the distal screws are applied to the plate and the compression fixture removed. On the ulna from the contralateral limb, shortening was carried out using a standard, AO 3.5 mm, 7-hole dynamic compression plate following a transverse osteotomy.

After the ulnas were stabilized with the above techniques five pairs were

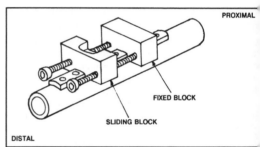

Figure 1a - The screws that hold the cutting guide, align th screws automatically for the plate in the same holes for th final position.

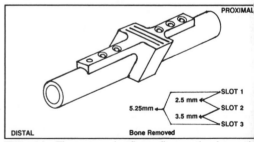

Figure 1 b - The compression fixture fits over the plate so th the final coaptation and compression is precisely controlle

ated for three-point bending and five pairs for torsion testing. For the three-point bend test, the
ratus was placed in the MTS servohydraulic testing system and subjected to a constant displacement rate
mm/sec within the elastic range in the medial-lateral plane in apex-radial bending. The load-
acement curve was recorded and the stiffness determined. The specimen was then tested to failure in
nterior-posterior plane in apex volar bending, using a constant displacement rate of 1 mm/sec.

For the torsion test, the ulna distal to the plate fixation, was potted in methylmethacrylate cement in
ure which incorporated a lever arm. The ulna was then placed in the MTS testing system and the lever
subjected to a force couple and rotated within the elastic range. The torque-rotation curve was recorded
he stiffness and strength was determined.

Comparison of the results was based on the structural behavior of each specimen noting the mean
standard deviation of the load to yield, load to ultimate failure, and the slope of the load-displacement
for both types of fixation. Comparisons between groups was made by the student's t-test.

For the clinical portion of the study twenty-three patients underwent transverse ulnar shortening
tomies between 05/10/88 and 07/28/89. There were twelve females and eleven males averaging 33.3
old (16-52). Indications for surgery were: triangular fibrocartilage tear (9), distal radial ulnar radial
joint incongruity (4), ulnocarpal impingement (6), lunotriquetral tears (2), and ulnar capsular tears (2).

A 3-5 mm. free-hand osteotomy was made 3/4 through the bone using a hand held saw. An external
ression device was then secured to the plate distallly while the proximal portion of the plate was firmly
in position with the two screws into the ulna. The osteotomy was then completed with the cutting of the
ior portion of each cut and removing the intervening bone segment. By tightening the horizontal
ded screws of the compression device the osteotomy was closed and the distal plate attacdhed to the
with 3 screws. The compression device was then removed after compression was accomplished and the
was affixed to the bone with standard 3.5 cortical screws.

Upon preliminary review of the prolonged healing time in the transverse osteotomy series, seventeen
nts underwent an oblique ulnar shortening osteotomy between 09/22/89 and 08/16/90. There were
females and fourteen males averaging 38.3 years old (range 19-55). Indications for surgery were:
gular fibrocartilage tears (11), ulnocarpal impingement (3), ulnar capsular tear (1), and lunotriquetral
(6).

Following the same operative approach as the transverse osteotomy, the oblique cutting guide from
ROS system* was firmly attached to the ulna with 3.5 mm cortical screws (Figure 1). A sagittal saw was
used to remove a 2.5 to 3.5 mm segment of
. The cutting guide was then replaced with the
alized slotted plate and compression fixture as in
ransverse osteotomy description above. After the
ends were reduced with the compression
ratus, a 2.7 mm interfragmentary lag screw was
ted across the osteotomy. The two distal screws
then drilled and applied, the compression-
action device was removed and the two holes
filled with the cortical screws to complete the
on.

In both groups of patients, a long-arm sugar
splint was applied at surgery and converted to a
-arm cast at the first post-surgical follow-up. At
month post-surgery, the long-arm cast was
ged to a short-arm cast which was subsequently
wed by the application of a removable splint for
er casting until fracture healing was confirmed.
ographs were taken at the first post-operative

ray Corporation, Arnprior, Ontario, Canada

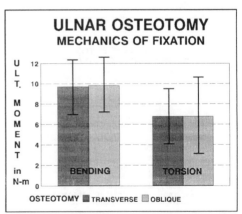

ULNAR OSTEOTOMY
MECHANICS OF FIXATION

Figure 2 b - Strength comparisons in bending showed no differences. (Bars are mean values, brackets are standard deviations).

visit at 10-14 days post-surgery and at four week intervals thereafter until bony union was obtained.

RESULTS:

Results of the laboratory testing comparing the three-point bend and torsion tests are shown in Figure 2. The oblique osteotomy fixation could not be statistically separated in ultimate moment or in structural stiffness from the transverse osteotomy fixation in either of the bending tests. This is in spite of the fact that the prototype slotted plate was only 54% as rigid as the standard 3.5 DCP plate as measured by ASTM four-point bending test (ASTM 383). However, the oblique osteotomy was statistically significantly stiffer in torsion than the transverse osteotomy at a significance level of P < .04.

Results of the clinical evaluation are based upon follow-up of all patients until healing was established, with one exception in a transverse osteotomy case which resulted in nonunion. Radiographic healing was defined as trabecular bone bridging across the osteotomy coupled with blurring of the cortical margins of the osteotomy. The same criteria were used to analyze the healing time of both oblique and transverse osteotomy groups. Twenty-two of the patients healed with transverse osteotomy at an average of 20.6 weeks post surgery (range 11-32 weeks). One patient's

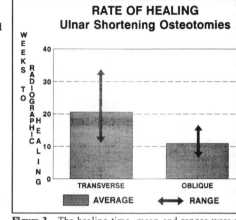

Figure 3 - The healing time mean and ranges were v different for the transvers vs. oblique osteotomies.

transverse osteotomy was declared a nonunion at forty weeks despite external electrical stimulation treatm for ten weeks. In contrast, the oblique osteotomy group healed in a substantially shorter 10.9 weeks avera (range 7-17). There were no nonunions in the oblique osteotomy group.

DISCUSSION:

The choice of apex-volar and apex-radial bending and axial torsion is based upon the author's fee

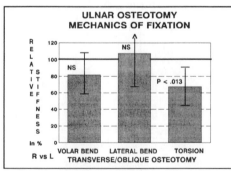

Figure 2 a - Stiffness was statistically significantly different only for torsion. (Bars are mean values, brackets are standard deviations).

of a need to measure multiple planes of loading b a lack of good clinical evidence that any particular mode is most responsible for mechanical failures clinically. It is easy to justify apex-radial loading since many injuries occur in this mode of loading and direct loading in this mode occurs when one rests one's arms on most surfaces, (a common posture for many activities of daily living). The n "worst" condition of loading is out of plane to the plate[6] which creates rigidity and strength proxima 1/6 of that when loading the plate in a tension ba mode. Also, because of the tethering effect of the interosseous membering there seems to be little chance that the ulna could be loaded away from t radius so that the plate would act in a tension ban mode, therefore, this mode of loading was not tested. Axial torsion was included because of the torsion of the ulna during pronosupination of the forearm.

The ulnas used for this study were fixed in formalin and, therefore, had altered rigidity and resilience m what one would expect from fresh human bones. However, work by other investigators has indicated t the strength of cortical and trabecular bone fixed in formalin is not significantly altered from that of mal moistened bone.[8] Coupling this with the availability of formalin fixed bone, the fact that the study s designed to be an internally controlled, comparative study, only the relative fixation with each technique s compared (rather than the absolute numbers of the strength of fixation), the investigators felt that this del was adequate and fair for assessing the parameters measured.

For the clinical portion of this study it is recognized by the authors that it is difficult to identify cisely the date in which radiographic healing has occurred. Every effort was made to apply the same eria of fracture healing to both the transverse and oblique osteotomy group. It is not possible to apply ical criteria, such as pain or tenderness, along the osteotomy surface to determine the presence or ence of clinical healing as in closed treatment.[14]. This is clearly demonstrated by the patient who tinues to complain of pain over the subcutaneous border of the ulna when the osteotomy surfaces have g since ceased to be present radiographically. The sensitivity is usually relieved with removal of the plate er local anesthesia and is unrelated to the state of healing of the osteotomy in most cases (possibly ated to the bulk of the hardware). Also it must be noted that this subjective evaluation of healing was not ried out in a blind fashion by an independent observer, which could introduce bias into the study.

It should be stressed that it is not the one nonunion in the transverse osteotomy group of the study t prompted the use of the oblique osteotomy, but rather the excessively long healing time of the transverse eotomy. Based on the disconcerting data from the transverse osteotomy, the first author decided to ndon the transverse osteotomy in favor of the oblique osteotomy system in September, 1989. The greatly tened healing time of the oblique osteotomy which averaged 10.9 weeks, as presented in the study, ports the decision to abandon the transverse osteotomy of the ulna although it is not clear which factors responsible for this difference. Improved healing time in the oblique osteotomy group may be partly ibutable to the 40% increase in surface area of the 45° oblique osteotomy. Additionally, the rfragmentary lag screw placement which is made possible by the oblique osteotomy improves the npression at the osteotomy healing surface and increases the rigidity of the fixation of the construct. Still it st be noted that the clinical significance of mechanical strength and stiffness are unknown, and at best, culative. For instance, a rigid device with poor co-aptation (i.e. the transverse osteotomy with a large te) might be more rigid in bending than a more compliant plate achieving better co-aptation (i.e. the ique osteotomy), but the micromotion at the osteotomy sight could be less with the more compliant plate to improved co-aptation. It is the micromotion at the osteotomy site that probably delays healing the st according to tissue strain theories. While the transverse osteotomy group did not have an rfragmentary lag screw, it is generally accepted that placement of such a screw is technically demanding may, in fact, have a tendency to distract rather than compress the transverse osteotomy surfaces. This erence in healing time may also be related to the use of a less-rigid plate, and/or the oblique osteotomy, wing more stress to pass through the healing bone. Since the groups were done in series rather than allel, the learning curve of instrument use may have influenced the clinical results.

From the viewpoint of facilitating the surgical technique, the interfragmentary lag screw has the antage of "locking" the bone ends together after oblique osteotomy has been approximated, improving co-ation. This permits removal of the compression device without loss of bony opposition. This problem urred in the transverse osteotomy procedures upon removal of the compression device. The natural curve he bone against the "straight" plate caused the bone and plate to separate and the cortex opposite to the te to gap at the osteotomy site.

The use of the precision cutting and positioning guide in this study to create the oblique osteotomy bles the surgeon to remove a pre-determined amount of bone and to assure nearly perfect co-aptation of bone ends[11, 12]. The precision cutting guide allows the saw cuts to remain exactly parallel and to precisely ermine the amount of bone to be removed. It is acknowledged that the ability to perform parallel saw s in exceedingly difficult to obtain with a free-hand technique. The two blade technique described by edman[5], attempts to produce two free-hand parallel osteotomy surfaces. However, even with the use of a r, the surgeon, no matter how careful he or she might be, cannot accurately predict the exact amount of e to be removed. In re-approximation of the bone ends, malrotation may occur without visual appreciation at the osteotomy site. By using the same blade in this precision system, the surgeon is virtually assured of the accuracy of the osteotomy thickness. As a point of interest, with the blade designed for this systems, each saw blade removes .78 mm., or a total of 1.56 mm. with two saw cuts. It is obvious that the cut or step cut osteotomy faces the same obstacles of determining the amount of bone removed and the difficulty in precisely co-apting the bone surfaces. If these were as easy as some have claimed, this would have become the standard treatment since its introduction and association with plate fixation in 1974.[1]

It becomes clear that the precision of the oblique osteotomy obtained by this system is not likely to be attained by free-handing two oblique saw cuts no matter how skilled the surgeon. Cantero's use of the double Stryker blade is a method to produce two parallel cuts at a fixed distance. However, this technique has not been adopted since its inception in 1977.[2] To date, no surgical system has been available which allows the surgeon to reliably and predictably remove a specified amount of bone and then to apply easily a compression plate and interfragmentary screw in the performance of an oblique shortening osteotomy of the ulna.

The reproducibility, speed, and ease of this surgical procedure along with the shortened healing time make this system an attractive alternative to the present hand held technique. Since this study was completed, a drill and tap guide, for the interfragmentary screw at 22° relative to the osteotomy, has been added. This additional equipment adds to the sophistication and precision of the system. It should be noted that the increased stability achieved with this system has now prompted a more cavalier approach in post operative protection since this study was completed. In many instances, a removable orthoplast splint is all that is needed for post-operative protection. This less cumbersome immobilization makes the procedure more tolerable without jeopardizing osteotomy healing. It is anticipated that this study will prompt the use similar precision cutting guides, compression devices, and specialized plates for the shortening osteotomies other long bones in the body.

REFERENCES:

[1]   Cantero J: Re-establishment of supination by ulnar shortening in the sequelae of Colles' fractures (new technique). [French] Rev Med Acc, Vol. 67, 1974, p 135.

[2]   Cantero J: Shortening of the ulna in the sequelae of fractures of the distal radial extremity. (French) Ann de Chir, Vol. 1, 1977, pp 330-4

[3]   Darrow JC, Linsheid RL, Dobyns JH, Mann JM III, Wood MB, Beckenbaugh RD: Distal ulnar recession for disorders of the distal radioulnar joint. J Hand Surg, Vol. 10, 1985, pp 482-91

[4]   Faupel L: Indications and results in shortening osteotomy of the ulna. Unfallchir, Vol. 10, No. 5, 1984, pp 250-3

[5]   Friedman S, Palmar A: The ulnar impaction syndrome. Hand Clin, Vol. 7, 1991, pp 295-310

[6]   Lindahl O: The rigidity of fracture immobilization plates. Acta Orthop Scand, Vol. 38, 1967, p 10

[7]   Linsheid RL: Ulnar lengthening and shortening. Hand Clin, Vol. 3, No. 1, 1987, pp 69-79

[8]   McElhaney JH, Fogle J, Byars E, Weaver G: Effect of embalming on the mechanical properties of beef bone. J. Appl Psysio, Vol. 19, No. 6, 1964, pp 1234-6

[9]   Milch H: Cuff resection of the ulna for malunited Colles' fracture. J Bone Joint Surg, Vol. 39A, 1941, pp 311-3

[10]   Minami A, Toshihiko O, Minami M: Treatment of distal radioulnar disorders. J Hand Surg, Vol. 12A, 1987, pp 189-196

[11]   Rayhack J: Ulnar impaction syndrome: treatment by precision oblique ulnar shortening. Techniques Orthop, Vol. 7, 1992, pp 49-57

[12]   Rayhack J: Video Journal of Orthopaedics Vol. 7, 1992, p 2

[13]   Ruby L: American Society for Surgery of the Hand Correspondence Newsletter 1990-3.

[14]   Zych GA, Latta LL, Zagorski JB: Treatment of isolated ulnar shaft fractures with prefabricated fracture brace. Clin Orthop, Vol. 219, 1987, pp 88-94

John Gray Seiler, III,[1] Jesse B. Jupiter, Michael Miller, Mary Jo Albert, and Melton Doxey

THE 3.5 MILLIMETER LIMITED CONTACT DYNAMIC COMPRESSION PLATE: A PRELIMINARY REPORT OF TECHNICAL ADVANTAGES

REFERENCE: Seiler, J. G., III, Jupiter, J. B., Miller, M., Albert, M., and Doxey, M., **"The 3.5 Millimeter Limited Contact Dynamic Compression Plate: A Preliminary Report of Technical Advantages,"** Clinical and Laboratory Performance of Bone Plates, ASTM STP 1217, J. Paul Harvey and Robert F. Games, Eds., American Society for Testing and Materials, Philadelphia, 1994.

ABSTRACT: A preliminary, prospective, multicenter study using the 3.5 mm low contact dynamic compression plate (LCDCP) for traumatic and reconstructive problems in the upper extremity skeleton is presented. Over a 13-month period in three institutions, 26 plates were implanted in 21 patients. Twelve were male and 9 female, with an average age of 26 years. Eleven LCDCP were used for acute fractures. Fifteen plates were used in reconstructions, including nonunions; radial osteotomies; and wrist arthrodeses. Twelve were stainless steel and 14 titanium. Plate lengths ranged from 6 holes to 10 holes. Multi-directional contouring was required in 6 cases. Obliquely placed 3.5 mm design "shaft" lag screws were used in 2 cases. In 4 cases, the plate design permitted compression in 2 opposing directions along the longitudinal axis of the bone. In one case, the newer hole design allowed placement of an oblique lag screw at a 40-degree angle to the plate. All patients were treated with a functional aftercare program. Radiographic and clinical union was achieved within 3 months in each case. There were no immediate or late postoperative problems. Functional limb recovery was noted in each case. One patient had plate removal 6 months post wrist arthrodesis due to extensor tendon inflammation. The plate was securely fixed. Microscopic sections of zones of contact and non-contact clearly demonstrated increased osteoporosis in the zones of plate contact. This experience supports the fact that with the LCDCP internal fixation is secure, plate design allows easier 3-dimensional contouring, and screw placement is facilitated.

KEY WORDS: Dynamic compression plating, fracture fixation, upper extremity

---

[1]Assistant professor of orthopaedic surgery, Department of Orthopaedic Surgery, The Emory Clinic, 1365 Clifton Road, N.E., Atlanta, GA 30322.

Introduction

The application of compression plates has become the most common method of treatment for certain fractures and nonunions of the tubular bones of the upper extremity. Commonly available dynamic compression plates have certain design characteristics which may limit their optimal intraoperative application. Difficulty in multi-planar contouring, a solid center section and limited ability to insert interfragmental lag screws through the plates are all limitations of currently available plating systems. Recently, a new type of dynamic compression plate, the limited contact dynamic compression plate, has been introduced to facilitate intraoperative application and to lessen cortical ischemia from plate application.

Recent basic science studies regarding the bone plate interface following the plating of fractures have focused on histologic changes and concluded the cortical contact by the plate has a significant effect on the development of cortical porosity (1, 2). Perren, et al., in an evaluation of platings of different materials, found that the single most important factor influencing cortical porosity was the amount of plate-bone interface (1). Their studies using in vivo techniques of cortical blood flow assessment have shown that a significant factor in the development of local porosity is a transient period of ischemia in the area beneath the plate. Experimental studies evaluating plates with limited cortical contact areas have shown that these new plate designs caused less cortical ischemia and a lower magnitude of reactive hyperemia in the cortical bone beneath the plate (2). Clinically, increased cortical density may be a substantial benefit at the time of plate removal. Increased torsional rigidity of the bone secondary to improved cortical strength may be hypothesized to contribute to a lower refracture rate after these plates have been removed.

The purpose of this study is to report a prospective clinical evaluation of a 3.5 millimeter limited contact dynamic compression plate for the treatment of traumatic and reconstructive problems of the upper extremity.

Materials and Methods

Beginning in September of 1990 a prospective study was begun at the Grady Memorial Hospital and the Massachusetts General Hospital to evaluate limited contact dynamic compression plates (LCDCP) for treatment of upper extremity fractures and reconstructive operations. All patients admitted to the services of the senior authors (JGS, JJ, MM, MJA) with closed diaphyseal forearm fractures or for correction of upper extremity skeletal deformities were considered as candidates for this study. Twenty-six plates have been implanted in 21 patients since that time. There were 12 men and 9 women. All patients were skeletally mature. Eleven plates have been placed for the treatment of acute diaphyseal forearm fracture and 15 plates have been inserted for upper extremity reconstructions.   Twelve plates were composed of 316L stainless steel and 14 were composed of a commercially pure titanium.   Emory investigators implanted stainless steel plates while Massachusetts General Hospital investigators used titanium plates. Plate lengths ranged from six to ten holes.   All plates were inserted using standard compression plating techniques. A specialized drill guide was used for   the insertion of compression screws through the LCDCP.

The limited contact dynamic compression plate (Synthes, Paoli,   Pa) design differs from the standard dynamic compression plate in that there is less cortical contact between the plate and the underlying bone.   Oblique under-cutting of the plate in the area of the screw hole limits the cross sectional area applied to the bone. The screw holes for the LCDCP are designed to allow compression through the plate in either direction and are evenly spaced along the plate. Elimination of the solid middle section of the plate increases the surgeon's ability to apply the plate to complex bones. The bending stiffness and torsional stiffness of the plate are not significantly different from the standard dynamic compression plate (3).   The design of the LCDCP allows the insertion of inter-fragmental lag screws through the plate inclined to 40 degrees, twice as much as can be achieved through the standard dynamic compression plate.

Results

All patients were followed by the authors until radiographic and/or clinical union occurred.   Radiographic union was seen in all patients in this series by three months postoperatively.   Radiographic union was defined as evidence of bridging trabecular bone.   Often in fractures plated anatomically the bone healed with primary bone union and the specific time of radiographic union was difficult to document. In these situations, clinical assessment was relied on to assess union.   In several cases the design of the plate offered intraoperative advantages.   In two cases a very oblique lag screw was able to be placed through the plate which would not have been possible with standard dynamic compression plates.   Complex multi-directional plate contouring was necessary for the application of six plates. The LCDC plates were able to be quickly and smoothly contoured for these complex applications. Further, for the treatment of clavicular nonunion a tricortical autogenous iliac crest graft was inserted as an interpositional graft to restore clavicular length.   In these situations the design of the plate allowed the surgeon to compress the intercalated segment from both sides of the nonunion.

A single plate has been removed one year after wrist arthrodesis.   Intraoperatively, the plate was found to be firmly fixed with minimal surrounding cortical reaction.   At the time of removal bone biopsies were harvested from areas of direct plate contact and from the areas of low contact but beneath the plate. Independent blinded histological evaluation of these specimens showed diminished osteoporosis beneath the areas of limited contact as compared to the areas of direct contact.

There were no wound infections or deaths in this series. One case of a distal third radius fracture was complicated by the formation of a radio-ulnar synostosis.

Discussion

Historically, Hansmann is often credited with being the first to use plates and screws for the fixation of fractures (4). In 1892, Sir William Arbuthnot Lane presented a similar approach to the treatment of tibia fractures by suggesting that operative open reduction and the application of internal fixation could be safely performed and would hasten a patient's recovery (5, 6). Sir Henry Platt, in his treatise on modern trends in orthopedics, recognized the importance of anatomical reduction of the fracture fragments and fixation sufficient to allow early adjacent joint mobilization (7). In separate reports both Key and Charnley reported increased success in arthrodesis performed with compression methods (8, 9). In 1949, Danis reported the first clinical review of fractures treated with a prototype compression plate (10). His system, the "coapteur," placed a screw at the end of the plate directed along the axis of the plate which when engaged pulled the opposite fragment towards the screw. Eggers noting the problems of nonunion and fatigue failure of plate fixation with fractures plated in distraction proposed the use of a slotted plate with screws inserted appropriately through the slots fixing the bone but allowing dynamic axial compression through the slots (11). Bagby, et al., in 1958, detailed a new "collision" plate which allowed compression of small gaps through the plate by tightening screws against a vertical screw hole (12). Simultaneously, the Arbeitgemeinschaft fur Osteosynthesesfragen (AO) group introduced a system of implants which improved the options for the plating of fractures. In 1970 Allgower and Perren reported the "dynamic compression plate" (DCP) as a method for providing rigid internal fixation (13). The design of the screw holes called for a ramp at the margin of the side of the hole which allowed increased compression to be applied through the plate.

Since that time, compression plating has become a common method employed to treat fractures and reconstructive problems of the upper extremity. Because of its design, the standard dynamic compression plate has been difficult to apply to bones with complex contours. In our series, The LCDCP was technically easier to apply to bones requiring multiplanar bending. Additionally, lag screws were able to be inserted through the plate at increased angles relative to the plate. Because of these design modifications the LCDCP was easier to apply for complex plating applications, such as the treatment of clavicular nonunions. In addition there were several hands

on advantages in application.   The plate is easily and
smoothly contoured. Even in cases requiring multidirectional
bending the plate was able to be quickly and satisfactorily
shaped for implantation. This may be secondary to the more
uniform stiffness along the plate that is associated with the
undercutting of the screw holes and uniform distribution of
the screw holes.   The newer design of screw hole allowed for
insertion of very oblique lag screws which could not have been
placed through a standard 3.5 millimeter dynamic compression
plate.   In the treatment of nonunions with intercalated
segment bone grafts the plate design allows compression in
both directions across the graft. Finally, the uniformity of
screw   hole   placement   along   the   plate   facilitates
intraoperative plate adjustments during implantation.

Uhthoff described the cortical changes that occur in
response to long bone plating (14, 15). He noted significant
cortical osteopenia and a reduction in shaft caliber beneath
DCP implants applied to long bones which was histologically
characterized by the presence of woven bone beneath the site
of   plate   application.   Finally,   these   histologic   and
radiographic changes were reversible after plate removal.
Interestingly, these changes seemed more pronounced in bones
internally   fixed   with   316L   stainless   steel   implants   as
compared to titanium plates.

The problem of refracture following plate removal is well
described. Deluca et al reported refractures in 7/67 forearms
following implant removal (16). Experimental studies have
suggested that the cause of refracture is diminished torsional
rigidity of the bone secondary to cortical porosis and the
presence of empty screw holes which function as stress
raisers. Recent experimental data has shown that the LCDCP
design causes less disturbance of cortical blood flow at the
time of application and is associated with a lower magnitude
of peak reperfusion and osteoporosis at eight and twelve weeks
postoperatively (2).   The increased cortical thickness
observed in bones plated with the LCDCP may improve torsional
rigidity following plate removal and lessen the chance of
fracture following plate removal.

The results of this preliminary report show satisfactory
rates of fracture union and no complications related to the
plating.   In this series both stainless steel and titanium
plates were inserted. In terms of achieving fracture union
both materials performed satisfactorily. This correlates with
the results of Holzach and Matter who showed no clinical
difference between the two plate materials in a trial of 256
consecutive tibia fractures treated by plating (17).   The
titanium plates are somewhat easier to contour but require
increased attention to detail at the time of insertion as the
screws are more easily sheared off at the junction between the
screw thread and the head. As of yet only one implant has
been removed in this series and in this patient, histologic
examination did show less cortical porosity in the areas of
cortex protected by the plate.

To address the clinical significance of improved cortical bone perfusion beneath the plate, a large prospective randomized trial will be necessary.

References

1. Perren, S.M., Cordey, J., Rahn, B.A., Gauthier, E., Schneider, E.: Early Temporary Porosis of Bone Induced by Internal Fixation Implants: A Reaction to Necrosis, not to Stress Protection. Clinical Orthopaedics and Related Res. 232: 139-151, 1988.

2. Swiontkowski, M.F., Senft, D., Taylor, S., Agnew S.G., Santoro, V.: Plate Design has an Effect on Cortical Bone Perfusion. Proceedings of the Orthopaedic Research Society. 66, 1991.

3. Gasser, B., Perren, S.M., Schneider, E.: Parametric Numerical Design Optimization of Internal Fixation Plates. Presented at 7th Meeting of the European Society of Biomechanics. Aarhus, Denmark, 1990.

4. Mears, D.C.: Materials and Orthopaedic Surgery. Baltimore, Williams & Wilkins, 1979.

5. Lane, W.A.: The Operative Treatment of Fractures. 2nd Edition, London Medical Publishing, 1914.

6. Lane, W.A.: The Direct Fixation of Fractures (abstract). Transactions of Clinical Society London 27: 167, 1894.

7. Platt, H.: Modern Trends in Orthopaedic Surgery. Medical Book Department of Harper and Brothers. 29-33, 1950.

8. Charnley, J.C.: Positive Pressure in Arthrodesis of the Knee Joint. Journal of Bone and Joint Surgery 30-B: 478-486, 1948.

9. Key, J.A.: Positive Pressure in Arthrodesis for Tuberculosis of the Knee Joint. Southern Med J 25: 909-915, 1932.

10. Danis, R.: Theorie et practique de l'osteosythese. Paris, Masson, 1949.

11. Eggers, G.W.: Internal Contact Splint. Journal of Bone and Joint Surgery 30A, 40-52, 1948.

12. Bagby, G.W., Janes, J.M.: The Effect of Compression Plates on the Rate of Fracture Healing Using a Special Plate. Am J Surg 95: 761-771, 1958.

13. Allgower, M., Perren, S., Matter, P.:   A New Plate
     Design: The Dynamic Compression Plate. Injury 2: 40-47,
     1970.

14. Uhthoff, H.K., Dubuc, F.L.: Bone Structure Changes in the
     Dog Under Rigid Internal Fixation. Clinical Orthopaedics
     and Related Research. 81: 165-170, 1971.

15. Uhthoff, H.K., Bardos, D.I., Liskova-Kiar M.:   The
     Advantages of Titanium Alloy Over Stainless Steel Plates
     for the Internal Fixation of Fractures: An Experimental
     Study in Dogs. Journal of Bone and Joint Surgery 63B:
     427-434, 1981.

16. DeLuca, P.A., Lindsey, R.W., Ruwe, P.A.: Refracture of
     Bones of the Forearm after the Removal of Compression
     Plates. Journal of Bone and Joint Surgery 70A: 1372-1376,
     1988.

17. Holzach, P., Matter, P.: The Comparison of Steel and
     Titanium Dynamic Compression Plates Used for Internal
     Fixation of 256 Fractures of the Tibia. Injury 10:
     120-123, 1978.

6-24-94